LIMITLESS

....

A 300-MILE RUN TO PROVE THAT
ANYTHING IS POSSIBLE

JUSTIN LEVINE

Justin Levine/Limitless
Printed in the United States of America

Limitless/ Justin Levine. -- 1st ed.

ISBN 978-0-692-59689-0 Print Edition

CONTENTS

To my wife, Stephanie, and two daughters, JoJo and Bobbi

You are the reason I do everything.

"Determination is stronger than weakness."

PREFACE

....

It was, for all practical purposes, a "normal" Tuesday morning. The date was January 29, 2013—a date I'll never forget as long as I live.

I was in a group training session at the fitness center I own when the phone rang. Normally, the receptionist would have taken a message. Not this time. It was my wife's obstetrician. He needed to talk to me. NOW.

Stephanie was thirty-five weeks pregnant; her due date was just eighteen days away and the excitement of our second child entering the world was dynamic beyond words.

I knew Stephanie was scheduled for a routine checkup that morning, not an occasion normally warranting a phone call from the doctor, not unless something was wrong, or, in this case, terribly, tragically wrong.

I remember his voice more than his exact words. It was that ominous mixture of subdued and serious, and I could feel a hole opening up in the pit of my stomach. When he delivered the words, " . . . we lost her heart rate . . . I'm so sorry . . . she died . . ." I felt a part of my world crack open and crumble right before my eyes.

I hung up the phone feeling numb and powerless. Shock and disbelief swept over me like a tidal wave; my legs gave way, and I dropped into the nearest chair. Then I pictured my wife, alone in that office, alone with her own disbelief, and I had to get to her.

I don't remember leaving the gym. I remember gripping the wheel of my car and a myriad of troubling questions scrambling in my head. "What could have possibly happened?" "Is this for sure?" "Did I hear the doctor correctly?" And then the most devastating of all: "Why?"

My biggest concern was for Stephanie. I have no memory of parking the car, only hurrying into the doctor's office and seeing the dismayed and saddened faces of the nurses; they told the whole story. I found Stephanie in an exam room, her face soaked with tears, and I took her tenderly in my arms. I have no idea how long we sat like that, crying and hugging, inconsolable in our grief.

After what seemed like an eternity, we finally collected our emotions enough to meet with the doctor. The trauma, I realized, had only begun. Our daughter was dead, but there was still the ordeal of giving birth to her. A stillbirth, the doctor called it. He advised an induced labor, and said the procedure wasn't something that could wait. He wanted us to be at the hospital later that afternoon.

Stephanie and I walked out of his office twenty minutes later, hurting as badly as two people possibly could.

We had an hour to hold our little one after her stillbirth. She was beyond beautiful. We named her Inspire. Yes, her life had ended in tragedy. No, we would never see her grow up, ride a bike, read a book, or fight with her sister. Yet the gifts she left proved an unexpected bounty. She would, like her name, inspire us. She would fire our determination to live the fullest life possible. In death, she would remind us never to give up hope, to strive for our goals even in the darkest hour, and to encourage not only one another, but all who came into our world. To inspire is to give strength, and that's what she left us: the strength to continue.

Two days later, we held a candlelight vigil at a friend's private lake in memory of our Inspire. Family and friends joined us in what was a somber, yet special night. As the sun set behind the lake and candles were raised in our daughter's honor, I hoped I would have the courage and strength to share the words I had written for Inspire the previous day:

We only get one life and we must take advantage of every single day we are on this beautiful Earth. Unfortunately, Inspire was unable to live in this life. But we can live with Inspire in all of us. Her beauty was like an angel. Her eyes closed were peaceful. She was absolutely perfect. Life will have many obstacles. How you handle your obstacles will define you as a human being. Find strength. Find resilience. Find hope. Find humility. Find optimism. Find your next step. There is no other way. Let's INSPIRE others to be positive, to be healthy, and to live life at a high level. Inspire will always be with us, maybe not in flesh, but in spirit. And the human spirit is one of the strongest forms of mankind.

———

This is the story of one man's race for inspiration. It began three months before Inspire was stillborn, and I realize now how much her spirit and presence impacted my desire to complete such an improbable—perhaps even insane—journey.

Running three hundred miles in four days was about finding my inner strength and defining my humanity. I was to learn along the way that determination is stronger than weakness. I was destined to find a way to drive a positive thought in the face of the most tragic and negative conditions. The physical, mental, and emotional distress of such an insane test of endurance was matched only by the determination and optimism that drove me onward, one stride at a time.

The journey was an epic one, and I came out of it a changed man.

It is my hope that sharing what I experienced in the pages of this book will change you in some positive way as well. It is my hope that you too will find determination in the toughest of times and joy in overcoming the obstacles that life invariably puts in our paths. It is my hope that you find a belief system that allows you to pursue your highest aspirations and focus on the positives in your life. It is my hope that you will set ambitious goals, create major action, and surround yourself with strong and positive relationships. It is my hope that my story will inspire you to push yourself past your comfort zone and into a world of possibilities.

The message is simple: anything is possible. Take one step at a time, run one mile at a time, and live a *LIMITLESS LIFE* one day at a time . . .

CHAPTER 1

....

BREAKING THE COMFORT ZONE

Saturday, October 19, 2012, 3:30 a.m.
Mile 265

Imagine running ten marathons in four days. There is a reason you're doing this, though the delirium and fatigue make it hard to remember exactly what that reason is.

Here I was, 265 miles into a three-hundred-mile endeavor that most people would have called slightly insane. I didn't see it that way. Pushing yourself to the limit is part of knowing yourself, knowing what you can be, knowing what you can achieve. That knowledge provides a platform for making a difference in the world in ways you didn't even know existed.

I wasn't alone. This wasn't about some solitary endeavor meant to prove my self-worth or my manhood; both were pretty well intact already. Breaking barriers is almost always about teamwork, and our team was the best. Hickey and Ira, my two pace runners, moved silently beside me. There was no rule against talking, thank goodness, and normally Hickey could run and carry on a conversation with the best of them. What he said didn't matter as much as knowing he was there. Even he was quiet at this stage of the trek.

A half dozen paces behind us, Jim pedaled his bike the way he always did, quietly and smoothly. He carried our food and fluids, but he also watched all three of us with an eagle eye. He watched for signs of distress, a term that was hard to define after 265 miles of pounding the pavement.

It was 3:30 Saturday morning. We were heading down Highway 1. I glimpsed a sign that read, "Welcome to Malibu County." With only thirty-five miles to go, the plan was to run through the night.

But there was a problem with that: confusion was beginning to set in. A lack of sleep and seemingly terminal exhaustion were giving birth to fits of delusion. For a guy who was completely sober, I felt pleasantly intoxicated. As we trotted along the dark and quiet highway, a universe of stars hovering above us, my eyelids became heavy. Right about then, I would have paid a king's ransom for a twenty-minute nap.

I saw our RV waiting for us up ahead—our home away from home—and we decided everyone could use some shut-eye. The entire crew was overextended, and we all needed to take a break. Hickey passed the word: we were shutting it down for 60 minutes. Sixty minutes didn't sound like much, but it would allow everyone to regain sufficient energy to finish what we'd started, an epic run that had the entire West Coast buzzing.

I didn't say a word. I hurried to the back of the RV, slipped off my shoes, and snuggled into my bed. You would have thought that after twenty-one straight hours of running, falling asleep would have been the easiest thing in world. Not so.

I had been running sixty-plus miles every day. Every joint in my body ached. Every muscle burned. My immune system had flamed out long ago. The physical wear and tear, however, was not the worst of it. Not by a long shot. It was the anxiety of knowing I had more miles yet to run that made falling asleep nearly impossible.

I may have nodded off for ten or fifteen minutes, but it hardly qualified as sleep. A thousand different thoughts were rumbling in my head, and I finally heard myself murmur, "Get up!"

I sat up. As much as I wanted to sleep, I knew I could not. My body was in complete overdrive. An endeavor like the one we'd undertaken pushed every part of my physiological system to the brink. I was near my limit. Anyone who has ever run a twenty-six-mile marathon will tell you that it forces the body to undergo tremendous physical duress. Here I was, in the middle of my tenth twenty-six-mile marathon.

I rolled out of my bed and lumbered into the RV's ultra-tiny bathroom. I looked in the mirror and saw a worn and tattered face, but worn and tattered didn't translate into doubt or discouragement. I stared into my eyes, and the eyes looking back at me were those of a determined competitor. I heard myself say, "Son of a bitch. Finish this."

I turned on the faucet, splashed some water on my face, and then gave myself a few slaps to wake up. I soaked my greasy hair, turned around, and closed the bathroom door behind me. I looked around the RV. Half my team was still sleeping. The other half had heard me shifting around, and they were just beginning to stir.

I felt bad. You didn't have to look too closely to see the depth of fatigue everyone felt. Every one of them had committed 100 percent to this project and were willingly sacrificing themselves without complaint to see it through. They had bought into my vision and made it their own. I could never truly express my gratitude.

Normally, I consider myself an upbeat and positive guy—I think most of the people I know would acknowledge that—but at that moment, I was fighting a wave of depression. Depression was the enemy, and there was only one antidote. Get moving.

After a quick bite to eat—a banana, a handful of nuts, and a candy bar—and sipping some hot coffee, I stumbled outside. My body was screaming. My feet were sore and swollen. My legs were beat up. My brain was beyond exhausted.

Yes, there was a well-defined goal hanging in the balance. And yes, I had no shortage of determination to keep moving forward. My body, however, was rebelling from the inside out, and the rebellion was getting the upper hand. Could I get my body to cooperate for another full marathon?

I stood by the side of the road and stared at the battlefield that lay ahead. Facing off on the front lines were my brain and my body. There was no heavy artillery in this battle. My body kept shouting, "*No!*" But my brain came back with an equally emphatic, "*Go!*"

I have no idea how long this internal tug-of-war went on. Suddenly, my younger brother Josh was standing behind me, putting his arm around my shoulders with the kind of loving tug only a supportive brother could offer.

Fatigue and mental anguish made it hard for me to understand what he was saying, but the sight of tears rolling down his face shook me to my core. He was crying. Crying hard.

Maybe he could see the world of hurt I was in; Josh was empathetic like that. And maybe he too felt the emotional overload of the journey we had undertaken. In either case, it hit me then, the intense amplitude of it all, this, the story of *Limitless* . . .

....

CHAPTER 2

"HAVE YOU ALWAYS BEEN LIKE THIS?"

Some time back, a local newspaper reporter opened his interview with me by asking, "Have you always been like this?"

This is the kind of question you get when you're planning an unprecedented three-hundred-mile run over a four-day span. Nonetheless, I had to stop and think about this for a moment. I bought some time by answering, "Have I always been like what?"

"Well, determined. Kind of crazy?" He chuckled.

"First time I've ever been asked that one," I told him. I didn't take offense at the question. Instead of addressing his "kind of crazy" question, I found myself talking about the roots of my determination, a gift from my loving and compassionate parents.

"They always believed in me," I said.

As far back as I can remember, my parents always encouraged me to give my all in every situation. They encouraged me to set goals and take the most determined approach possible to achieve them.

I remember doing just that at a very young age. When I was ten, our Little League team sold M&Ms to earn money for uniforms and equipment. It was a contest. The winning prize for the most M&Ms sold was a Super Nintendo. Yeah, I am definitely dating myself, but back then there wasn't much a kid wouldn't do for a Super Nintendo. I not only wanted to win, I wanted to win by a landslide. I told myself I would sell so many boxes of M&Ms that my competitors wouldn't have a prayer.

I stood in front of grocery stores for hours at a time asking anyone and everyone walking out of that store if they would contribute to my endeavor and made sure they knew how much our Little League team would benefit. I remember that either Mom or Dad was with me the entire time, both of them supporting my efforts 100 percent, just like they did all my entrepreneurial endeavors.

When I took on a morning paper route, delivering newspapers at 5:15 a.m., they encouraged me to be the best paperboy I could be. I can't tell you how many times my dad got up and ran the route with me; not because I needed the help, but just to show his support. If I wasn't on my bike, we'd run the route together, and that's probably where my love of running began.

I set a goal to "porch" every one of my customers' papers. It was a game, but it was also a challenge. At Christmas time, I gave each one of my customers a little gift of some kind; it was a token of thanks, but it was also a way of cementing my relationship with each of them. I was a businessman even then, I suppose.

I inherited my work ethic from my parents, as well. I saw them working hard every day, and I saw them taking pride in a job well done, even if it was a chore around the house.

"Be the best you can." I heard that many times. "Don't be afraid of a hard day's work and don't be afraid to fail once in a while." That was another well-learned lesson.

When it came to sports, it was my parents who believed in me first and foremost.

Physical size was not my greatest ally. At 5'5", I quickly realized that my heart and my drive needed to make up for the inches I did not have. What I did have, however, was the work ethic, discipline, and passion to do my best, three qualities that began as family traits and eventually turned into the personal values I have lived by ever since.

We didn't have a lot of fancy things growing up, but we had what we needed to be a happy family: love, compassion, and tolerance (and yes, a heavy dose of patience). I have two brothers and a sister. Jason is the oldest, followed by Elizabeth. Josh, who I introduced you to earlier, is the youngest. We were close growing up and are even closer now. I'm lucky in that regard; I know plenty of siblings who don't connect with each other and don't wish that on anyone.

My dad is a schoolteacher with forty years under his belt. He firmly believes that every child deserves the best education possible, and he continues to teach today. His hard work and passion are qualities I respect greatly and try to emulate. My mother is a devout Catholic and one of the most loving women you would ever meet. Church every Sunday was mandatory in our family. We all fought it at times, but Mom never gave in; we were going whether we like it or not. Our faith was not something she negotiated, and she liked church as a way of instilling strong values into our souls. Now, as a husband and father, I'm glad she didn't relent.

Over the years, my parents took in over forty foster kids. We treated each and every one of those kids like our own brothers and sisters. Mom and Dad may have demanded it in the beginning, but it taught us to love with an open heart, no matter what the circumstances. I would have to say that I still try to live by that mantra.

In my mid-twenties I was introduced to a Brian Tracy CD titled, *Eat That Frog*. It was an educational collection that talked at length about goal-setting strategies. Once I listened to it, a treasure chest of new ideas and endless possibilities opened for me, and I started diving into an array of personal-growth resources. My favorites are still Jim Rohn and Robin Sharma. Jim Rohn's *The Art of Exceptional Living* changed my life in many ways. I have listened to that CD at least twenty times from start to finish. My favorite quote states: *"Life doesn't get easier, you just get better."* I cannot tell you how important those eight words have been to me, especially in the tough times.

We all have our wish lists. Sometimes I wished for an easier life. Sometimes I wished for better weather or fewer problems. Sometimes I wished for more money or less conflict. But that's not how life works. *The Art of Exceptional Living* inspired me to take full responsibility for the things that I want in my life, and that is a priceless gift.

Robin Sharma is one of the world's foremost leadership experts and, like Jim Rohn, someone I respect highly. He says this on the subject of leadership: *"Leadership is about having unshakeable faith in your vision and unrelenting confidence in your power to make positive change happen."*

This powerful quote has taught me to be resilient even in the most difficult of times. It reinforces for me the fact that a quick-fix mindset is not the answer when it comes to pursuit of my goals. Creating a personal philosophy that incorporates Mr. Sharma's view of leadership has truly strengthened my personal growth over the past ten years, and reminds me that I can affect positive change if I'm willing to go the extra mile.

I learned early on that becoming a life student was well within my control. If I wanted to improve as a human being, I would have to work on the craft, and I was committed to doing that. If I wanted to become the man I desired to be, I would need to develop my own set of personal-growth tools, and I would need to implement strategies meant to reinforce positive behavior.

"Learn to work harder on yourself than you do your job," Jim Rohn likes to say, and I have to come to believe that working on my complete self creates a more well-rounded individual. This is not about perfection. I don't aspire to be perfect. All I can do is *strive every day to be a little better than I was yesterday.*

Even more than that, I believe we should embrace our imperfections. I think we are better as people if we embrace our individual flaws and faults and use them to our advantage. There is inspiration to be gained from our individual uniqueness. It runs in my veins and I'm sure it runs in yours.

The minute I feel like I am not moving forward, I find something to give me a jump-start, something that inspires me and pushes me forward. When stagnation sets in, I know a downward spiral is not far behind, and that is why I have never accepted the status quo. I am constantly challenging myself and always searching for personal improvement.

Some people view the drive for personal improvement as obsessive. Others see it as selfish. My view is quite the opposite: it is a necessity of life. If I am not taking full advantage of each day, of each minute, and each second, I am simply wasting time, and time goes far too fast to be wasted. I understand that each day is a small piece of my entire life. I live life on the edge. I strive for true potential. It's a journey I have committed to and committed to with vigor.

I fear not living to my ultimate potential. This fear is what gets me up in the mornings, ready to take on the day. This fear motivates me. It sparks a passion for living each day as if it were my last.

I have discovered the four essentials in our lives: health, relationships, time and financial wherewithal. I look at these four and want to maximize each with equal effort. One, I know, benefits the other. And I know that expending one to the detriment of another does not serve my personal development.

An integral part of this personal growth and development is the enthusiasm I draw on that drives me toward my goals. I believe that enthusiasm and drive are self-generated; you don't have to sit around and hope they appear out of the blue. This is how I live my life. It's also how I encourage others to live.

I have always been an athlete.

According to my parents, I was swinging a baseball bat and kicking around a soccer ball the moment I started walking. Athletics, I suppose, are a natural part of my genetic code. There wasn't a sport I wouldn't try when I was younger. Soccer, baseball, basketball, tennis, golf, swimming, football; you name it, I was willing to try it. Soccer and baseball were definitely my favorites. True, I was always the smallest kid on the field or court, but that did not matter. In fact, it motivated me. I believed in my abilities, and I wanted to prove that physical size didn't matter. Size, I came to realize early on, is no match for determination.

In high school, I discovered a natural talent for kicking a football. I was a freshman at the time and a member of freshman football team. One day the varsity punter missed practice, and the coach called my number. I had never kicked a football before, but I had been playing soccer since I was five, so kicking a ball of any kind came naturally. My first kick traveled a good forty yards and was a perfect spiral. The next went even farther and put a smile on my coach's face. He had me try a few kickoffs and field goals, and my career as a placekicker was effectively launched.

I was excited by this new and unexpected role, but I decided I didn't want to be just an average kicker. Knowing that practice makes perfect, I began kicking throughout the year. I kicked thousands of footballs. By the time I was a senior in high school, I was one of the top placekickers in California. The goal was to earn a scholarship and kick in college. In fact, it was the only option. After weighing a number of offers, I decided to attend the College of the Sequoias (COS), the local junior college. This gave me the opportunity to save money by living at home, attend a quality school, and continue my football career.

Football became my passion. Well, that and partying and chasing girls.

It was quite a sight. Here I was, standing 5'5", weighing no more than 145 pounds, and I was playing college football. I was like an ant among elephants. My best friends were the linemen, the big boys. Most of these guys were twice my weight and at least half a foot taller. Nonetheless, it was completely "normal" for me to be out there in my uniform acting like I belonged. At least I thought so. And my size didn't matter because I could kick the hell out of the ball, and I knew it.

After two years at COS, I earned a scholarship to New Mexico Highlands University (NMHU) in Las Vegas, New Mexico. During my first year at NMHU, I ranked as one of the top kickers in Division 2 football. After two years, I graduated at the top of my class with a degree in Human Performance and Sport. I was just as proud of that accomplishment as I was of my football accolades, and I knew my future hinged on my degree, not my kicking leg.

I confess that it wasn't all work and no play at NMHU. Like most college kids, I loved to party. What can I say? I liked having good time. My mindset could be summed up in six words: *anything worth doing is worth overdoing*. But drinking, smoking weed, and partying until all hours of the night are not ideal performance components, and the high life caused me to stray from my ultimate potential as a placekicker.

Fortunately, I found a mentor who had my best interests at heart. His name was Professor Dennis Francois. He was the first person who really talked with me man-to-man about goal setting and understanding my priorities. He liked to say, "What's most important to you? As soon as you know the answer to that question, your goals will fall into place."

Professor Francois got me back on track. Don't get me wrong; I still partied. I just shifted the high life down on my priority list. The idea was to handle the most important things first. Then I could go out and have a good time. Not a bad college philosophy, right? At least it worked for me.

I was in my junior year when I wrote down a list of goals I hoped to achieve over the next ten years, and I still have that well-traveled piece of paper. Looking back, I'm proud to say that I actually achieved every single one of those goals. Not because I am exceptionally gifted and super intelligent. I think it's because I'm an action taker. I think it's because I've been blessed with an extreme sense of determination. Do I sometimes drive myself crazy with this incessant need to push forward? Maybe a little. But I'd rather be active than idle. I'd rather be doing than watching. If I have an area of concern, it's probably not taking the time to appreciate a job well done or an obstacle overcome. I will say, however, that I am getting better at those.

With my college days winding down, I began applying to universities throughout the country looking for internships in fitness, sports marketing, or strength and conditioning. Notre Dame University called me, gave me a phone interview, and offered me a position.

After graduating from NMHU in August 2002, I moved to South Bend, Indiana for a one-year "Facilities/Fitness" internship. I gained a tremendous amount of experience managing a 72,000-square-foot recreation center. I also began kicking again. I regained my form. This led to tryouts for the Arena Football League, a stop at the NFL kicking combine, and opportunities at various kicking camps. I realized that landing a spot on a professional football team was extremely difficult. I also realized that if I really wanted to play football at the professional level, persistence was my primary ally. My ultimate goal was to kick in the NFL. As a reminder of this objective, I wore a thin rubber band around my wrist.

In the meantime, I started pursuing opportunities in the personal-trainer profession. I started with equipment assessments and exercise surveys at Notre Dame. Then I began training students and faculty. This led to my first taste at designing fitness and strength programs. I couldn't believe how much I loved being in the gym and helping people set fitness goals and finding the most effective workout regimen to achieve those goals. I had always been a people-person, and the profession fit me to a T.

After a year at Notre Dame, I moved back to California. I started offering personal training at a commercial gym. I continued kicking. I was twenty-three. Enjoying life came naturally. In 2004, I received a phone call from the Central Valley Coyotes Arena Football team. The Coyotes were a Division 2 team located close to my hometown. I got the call on a Monday, tried out and signed a contract on Tuesday, and I kicked in my first game the following Saturday. Some people might attribute it to fate, but I'm more apt to attribute it to hard work, hustle, and persistence.

I kicked for the Coyotes for one season and had a blast. I ended the year as one of the top placekickers in the league. For reasons I never fully understood, the Coyotes didn't re-sign me, and this turn of events proved to be both unfortunate and fortunate. Unfortunate because it was tough calling it a career; after all, football had been a big part of my life up until then. Fortunate because I have always managed to bounce back from disappointment quickly and realized there was no point in sulking. And fortunately, when one door closed another door opened.

Even while I was kicking for the Coyotes, I worked as a personal trainer at the Visalia Racquet Club in my hometown of Visalia, California. All the while, I was in the process of building my credentials and forging an expertise in the fitness industry. I loved showing up at the gym every day to train my clients. The club, in essence, allowed me to reinvent its personal training department, and things began to boom. Within twelve weeks, I had a completely full schedule. I worked my ass off and loved it. Up at 4:30 a.m., first client at 5:15 a.m., training sessions all day, last client at 7:00 p.m. I would be leaning on a piece of equipment just to stay up. I loved the profession. It became my life's work.

The opportunity to open my own fitness business became a reality in 2006. Over the previous year I had built a very solid relationship with the father of two kids I had been training at the club. He said that I had "changed his kids' lives." Furthermore, he told me that whenever I was ready to open my own fitness facility that he had an interest in being my private investor. I was as much in awe of his proposal as I was humbled by his faith in me. I am still humbled today.

It speaks to another important life lesson that has been instrumental throughout my life: build relationships. Building relationships is not about wanting something or expecting something from another person. It's about knowing that person "has your back" and that "you have his or her back." One thing I have certainly discovered: surrounding yourself with people that you trust and who support your mission is critical to becoming successful, both as a person and as a professional.

Without much actual understanding of the business world, I put together a very simple business plan and, with the help and support of my investor, opened California Fitness Academy (CFA) in August 2006.

To this day, I love what I do. I do not mind the 3:55 a.m. alarm clock or the twelve- to fifteen-hour workdays that business owner-ship brings. I do not mind the challenges or the criticism inherent in my position. No, it has not all been peaches and cream. There have been some tough times and there will continue to be. That's life. But the rewards of my profession outweigh any negatives.

My passion and obsession for living life to the fullest and help-ing others can sometimes ruffle feathers. I am, however, fine with going against the grain and challenging others to do the same. There is nothing wrong with feeling a little uncomfortable; in fact, that is when you know you're stretching your limitations. That discomfort is a sign of growth. I believe that unconditionally.

CFA started in a 2,400-square-foot facility with zero members and one employee: me. It was all about hustle and determination. Those two words (hustle and determination) have become natural traits of mine. They are now part of my DNA. There is no ques-tion that building a business from the ground up is a challenge. I remember any number of times during those first few years when I thought, *How the hell am I going to pay rent this month?* Well, I've never missed a rent check in eight years of business, and I can only attribute that to hustle and determination.

One of my primary goals over the years has been to provide a positive and uplifting environment for both my customers and employees. I can't see it being much fun if I don't.

I will admit, however, that there are some downsides to self-employment. As my wife will tell you, it's consuming. When I'm at home, I am thinking about business. When I'm on my bike, I am thinking about business. When I am with my family, I am think-ing about business. When I'm lying in bed at night, I am thinking about business.

California Fitness Academy is 6400 square feet. We have trained thousands of individuals from all walks of life. I truly believe that you can change the world by inspiring others to be great. I wanted a lifestyle that would support this notion. I've found it.

My community is very important to me, and I love giving back in any way I can. Over the past eight years, CFA has helped raise more than $50,000 for local nonprofit organizations and families in need. We organize charity boot camps and food drives. We hand out food to the homeless.

There is one story in particular that carries special meaning for me. I met five-year-old Aarin through a mutual friend and he is now my good buddy. In January 2013, Aarin was diagnosed with lymphoblastic leukemia, a rare form of blood cancer.

I was connected with Aarin and his family later that year, and I knew from the first moment how special this kid was and how full of life he was, even as he battled this disease. I knew from that first moment that I wanted to devise some kind of plan to raise money to help Aarin and his family with medical bills, travel, and hospital expenses. We decided on the spot that August would be Aarin Strong Month, and we encouraged the CFA community to donate in any way they could to support the cause.

The month culminated with an event we called the Aarin Strong Rep Challenge. The idea was that committed individuals would go out and get sponsors to give a certain amount of money for each repetition completed. The event raised close to $5,000. In total, we raised $8,500 the entire month.

What a life-awakening moment that experience was for me. When things don't go exactly as planned in my life, I think about Aarin and his struggles. Talk about perspective.

The amazing news is that Aarin's cancer is now in remission. This kid's courage and resiliency are truly inspiring. We can push through tough times if we have the right kind of mindset. We can battle through our obstacles and come out on the other side looking at life in a positive light, exactly as Aarin has done.

CHAPTER 3

······································

THE "ROAD" TO THE ENDURANCE LIFESTYLE

Growing up, I never considered myself a "runner." I would go out occasionally while I was in college and run five or six miles just to burn some calories and enjoy some quiet time. I certainly didn't know anything back then about triathlon training or living what I now call the "endurance lifestyle."

I had a friend in college who competed in a sprint triathlon one spring, and his participation and enthusiasm over the race struck a chord with me and motivated me to train for my first event. When my football career came to its unexpected ended, I switched gears and went right into basic triathlon training.

I completed my first race in 2005 at the Breath of Life Triathlon held in Ventura, California. It consisted of a 400-yard swim (in the ocean), a twelve-mile bike ride, and a three-mile run. I basically signed up on a whim. My approach was, "Why not?"

Looking back, I remember walking up to the transition area thinking, *Wow, there are some fit athletes here*. True, I was also fit, but in the sense of general fitness. It is, after all, a job requirement in my profession to look fit and stay healthy. But there is a difference between personal-trainer fit and endurance-sport fit. "Fit" in the triathlon sense does not mean you can bench press 250 pounds or squat three hundred pounds. It doesn't mean you look like a world-class body builder.

I learned quickly that triathlon fit meant that you could plunge into a lake or the ocean and swim with speed and energy, then go straight over to a bike and ride flat out, and without missing a beat get off your bike and run at a race-ready clip. Fit took on a new dimension in this sport. I showed up to my first event excited, eyes wide open, and slightly intimidated. I also showed up ready to see what I could do. Problem one: I had no wetsuit. Instead, I wore Under Armour underwear and proudly deemed it my "race suit." I had a heavy but serviceable road bike and plenty of guts. I even gave myself a Mohawk haircut as I "battled for war."

Humility quickly set in. I jumped into the fifty-five-degree ocean water and my lungs basically forgot how to breathe. I had one slightly coherent thought, *What was I thinking not wearing a wetsuit?* I was cold. Ok, I was freezing! As I was battling the ocean current and the crashing waves, I started thinking, *What the hell am I doing out here? This is miserable.*

Somehow I managed to get through it. Four hundred yards might not sound like much, but think about swimming four lengths of a football field in a perpetually moving sea. I shivered as I ran toward the transition area and continued to shiver as I put on my bike clothes. My mouth was so paralyzed by the cold I couldn't even manage a word, much less a smile, to the family and friends who had come to watch the event.

Eight miles later, I finally warmed up and gained some much-needed momentum for the final four miles of the bike segment of the race. I got off my bike feeling almost human again and hit the running stage of the race feeling strong.

Running has always been my strength and it was by far the strongest leg of my triathlon that day. I finished the event in one hour and thirty-five minutes. Had you asked me then, I probably would have proclaimed that my one and only triathlon. Safe to say I didn't really have that "good of a time." However, once the "I'm not sure if I like this sport" feeling wore off, I started thinking, *I want to get better at this sport. I want to excel at it.*

The speed of triathlon became my new endeavor. It was the first step toward a lifestyle dedicated to swimming, biking, and running. Training became a habit. Ok, it became an obsession, to be more accurate. I did not have any fancy gear or any of the latest equipment. Swim training began in a twelve-yard recreation pool. Bike training consisted of endless laps around a neighborhood park on an old mountain bike. Run training took me all over the city.

I made a fantastic discovery: I enjoyed triathlons because I loved pushing myself to my limits. The two went hand in hand. I also enjoyed it because there was always something new to work on and because the sport was so humbling.

I was not very good in the beginning. I was also not genetically gifted in this sport. But I knew that with hard work and determination I could improve and get faster. I planned family trips around triathlons. I trained come rain or shine, in hot weather and in cold.

From the outset, I looked at it as an investment, both in time and money, and I was fully invested.

Safe to say, I am who I am today because of my triathlon career. The sport taught me to be a better man. It taught me to push myself, even in the toughest of times. All along, a sense of great discipline was being formed, another important trait upon which I have built in my life. In fact, the word "discipline" is tattooed on my right leg. That is how important it is to me.

This habit of self-imposed and essentially gratifying discipline helped me create the mindset to believe that anything is possible.

After completing a number of triathlons—and meeting the personal "time" goals I set for each—I dove deep into the endurance world. Reading extensively on the subject, attending education workshops to further my knowledge, and attending coaching clinics on the subject all became part of my life.

My growing enthusiasm and interest level in triathlons pushed me to want to train with other like-minded individuals. Unfortunately, the triathlon community in Visalia was small at best.

I should start a club, I thought to myself. It was a glimmer of an idea. After talking to a good friend about triathlons and discussing the idea of starting a club, we put the idea out there to see how the community would respond. We set up a "club meeting" for any interested individuals. Our first "meeting" attracted four people. But the lack of attendance didn't matter to us. We enjoyed our conversations around the subject of triathlons and found fellowship among the few individuals in the club. Eventually four turned into ten, and ten turned into twenty. This would be the baby stage in the evolution of The Visalia Triathlon Club.

In 2007, The Visalia Triathlon Club became an official entity. Continued persistence, word of mouth, and constant education helped build the club over the years. What started out as a hobby became a major component in my life.

The Visalia Triathlon Club is now home to sixty-plus members. I am proud to be called "coach" by this group of motivated, positive, and upbeat individuals. I have made long-lasting and genuine friendships thanks to the people I have met through the sport. I am all about surrounding myself with like-minded, supportive, and positive people and the club has always been a prime outlet to make that happen.

Over the years, triathlon training and racing has become a lifestyle for me. On the morning of April 19, 2008, I competed in a local sprint triathlon and I took fourth place overall. That same evening Stephanie and I got married. I took first place that night!

Call me crazy, but training, racing, and improving in triathlons have long been ingrained in my life. Some guys play golf the morning of their wedding. I did a triathlon. So what!

Since that first event in 2005, I have competed in more than eighty different endurance events, from 5ks to sprint triathlons to my one and only Ironman competition. I have also coached and trained all levels of endurance athletes. Seeing others succeed in the sport is just as rewarding as my own individual accomplishments.

I have put on running workshops, nutrition clinics, and strength-training clinics. I have along the way also written for various national endurance and fitness websites. At the time of my first triathlon, I had no clue that I would develop into an experienced endurance athlete and run coach. I have built some of the finest friendships a man could ask for, and that is the most satisfying part of all.

Starting in 2007, I logged every one of my workouts. I use www.trainingpeaks.com as a tool to log, structure, and build my training regimen. Logging my workouts has been a vital tool to improving my performance, because I am able to look back at previous training days and races and analyze specific benchmarks. This directs my training and helps me evaluate my progress. In this log, I make notes on how I am feeling, the pace I set, and the mileage I completed.

Remember my mantra: *If it's worth doing, it's worth overdoing.*

These are some of my individual training and racing statistics since I began logging my training in 2007:

- Biking: 17,500 miles
- Running: 8,500 miles

- Swimming: 1,000,000 yards (Yes! One million yards in the pool)
- Half-marathon personal best: 1:22:45
- 5k best: 17:39
- 10k best: 37:50
- Half-Ironman best: 4 Hours 45 Minutes
- Ironman Arizona: 11 hours 10 minutes

I am not sharing these statistics as way of boasting about any particular achievement. In fact, these are not jaw-dropping numbers by any means. For me, these numbers are more than just times and mileage. They are pieces to the puzzle that make me the man I am today. Every mile, minute, or hour has been hard earned. There is no easy way to build endurance and there is no easy way to hit personal bests. It takes years of training. It takes dedication to the sport, great attention to healthy nutrition, and ample recovery.

When I began my love affair with endurance sports, I did not want to be average. I wanted to compete and perform at the best of my ability. I do not have some special DNA that makes me a natural endurance athlete. In fact, I am better suited for power sports like kicking a football or a soccer ball. But I made triathlons my lifestyle. With deep commitment and practice, I improved.

My triathlon lifestyle was just the beginning of something big in my life. More to come on that.

CHAPTER 4

....

IT WAS JUST AN IDEA

With an ambitious mind come outrageous ideas. I've always believed this.

The Limitless project started as a momentary glimpse, a passing thought.

I had just completed Ironman Arizona in November 2011. Just like I do with the athletes that I coach, I stopped and reevaluated the goal I had just achieved. Ironman training is a grueling process. It requires ten to twenty-five hours of training for at least four months to properly prepare for this ultra-distance event. Your body is taken to its limits during the training process. Training weeks are full of one-hundred-mile bike rides, twenty-mile runs, and torturously long swims. A normal weekend of Ironman training includes a Saturday bike ride somewhere between seventy to one hundred miles with a brick run (meaning right after the bike ride), followed on Sunday by a fifteen- to twenty- mile run.

Finishing IM Arizona was a huge accomplishment. But once I was done, I needed a break. I had spent the previous six years in the trenches of triathlon training, averaging at least twelve hours a week. I was burned out. The six weeks after Ironman included light, unstructured, and minimal training to allow my body and mind to recuperate after a grueling Ironman season. My first thought for the following season was to focus on shorter triathlons and to lay off the big training weeks. I wanted to focus on my family and business and allow my training to take a back seat. I was actually excited to design a program to improve my speed at shorter races like 10ks and sprint triathlons.

But if something is worth doing, why not overdo it, right? Here we go with my "all in" mentality.

The idea of a moderate training season dissipated after we spent the Christmas holiday that year with Stephanie's parents. During this five-day vacation, I took some time to just run. No watch, no structure, just whatever came to mind for that particular day. Luckily for me, my in-laws live in the mountains of Calaveras County in the small town of Arnold, California. With beautiful running trails and routes, it's a runner's paradise. The day before we were supposed to head home, I decided to make the trek from Arnold to Visalia on foot. I told Stephanie that I would start "running home" and she could pick me up along the road. The night before, I packed the truck and made sure everything was ready to go so Stephanie could just get in the truck with our daughter and drive. I took off just before sunrise; my watch read 6:15 a.m. She left four hours and twenty-two miles later and picked me up.

During that spur-of-the-moment run, I was struck with an epiphany. A light bulb went on halfway through the run, like a switch inside my head. The first whisper of a "big adventure" filled my head. I didn't really have any idea of what this "big adventure" would entail, but the seed had been planted.

I told Stephanie that it would be cool to "run to Los Angeles or something." She had every right to question my sanity, I suppose, but she didn't. This seed opening up inside me reignited the motivation I had found waning after the triathlon season ended. A voice inside me kept saying, "I believed I can do more. I believe I can accomplish something big."

More importantly, I wanted to inspire others.

But what would that "something big" be?

I am not sure what sparked this thought process, but I have always done my best thinking while I was running; well, at least some of my craziest thinking. Suddenly this idea of a long-distance run began to surface. But not just a marathon or an ultra-marathon—I wanted to put together a full-blown project.

That night I ran the longest distance I had run since the Ironman, another out-of-the-blue idea that I just had to act on. Oh, man! Let me tell you, my body was the victim of this crazy notion, and I was sore for days.

This thought of a full-blown project—something big—carried over into the new year. Out of nowhere, the idea of ultra-distance running became very intriguing to me. This was more than a little odd. Months before I had told my good friend and training partner, Eric Blain, just the opposite. I quote: "These ultra-distance events are not for me."

To this point, I had never even completed an official marathon. But something was pulling my interest toward the ultra-distance running world.

Forget the marathon. Let's just skip right to the ultra-distance, I jokingly thought.

There was something about the unknown of this very elite arena that sparked my interest. There is a mysterious characteristic to ultra-running. Despite all the preparation and training that goes into these runs, there are always deep and unfamiliar factors and obstacles that arise—almost spiritual moments—that ultra-runners have to face and overcome.

Ultra-runners have extraordinary strength of character and a strong mental capacity, and I wanted to explore their world. I also wanted to push my own personal limits. I wanted to see how far I could go. I wanted to grow not just as an athlete, but also as a human being. I wanted to find myself and look deep within my soul.

Ultra-distance running is characterized by distances over the traditional 26.2-mile marathon. Common ultra-running events are 50k (thirty-one miles), 80k (fifty miles), 100k (sixty-two miles) and 160k (one hundred miles).

Yes, there are crazy people out there who actually train and compete in one-hundred-mile running races! It was never for me. To this day, I still think that I am better off running half-marathons. Nonetheless, I started to dive into this ultra-distance world to get a glimpse of the lifestyle.

The word "limits" started to weigh on my brain, and I wanted to explore why some people decide to push their limits while others choose not to. So one Friday, after a long day at the gym, I came home and started surfing the Internet. I was led to some videos of Dean Karnazes and David Goggins, two of the most respected and well-known ultra-runners in the community. Awesome athletes! Dean had completed some unthinkable feats. Once, he ran 199 miles straight, without sleep. He ran fifty marathons in fifty consecutive days in fifty different states. He also trekked across the United States on foot. He completed the Badwater Ultra-Marathon—not once, but ten times. This extreme event is known as the "world's toughest road race," calling for athletes to run 135 miles in the most brutal conditions in the desert.

Who thinks of these remarkable feats of endurance? "Pushers" of human endurance, that's who. Just like David Goggins, another freak of endurance. This Navy Seal regularly competes in 100- to 150-mile ultra-marathon events. In 2013, he became the world record holder for the most pull-ups in twenty-four hours, busting out 4,030 repetitions in seventeen hours. Goggins pursues these physical challenges to raise money for the Special Operations Warrior Foundation, an organization that supports the families of fallen special-operations personnel.

"I train until the body is uncomfortable. That's truly when you know who you are," Goggins says.

As I watched the YouTube videos of these two ultra-athletes, I started thinking: *How far can I take myself? Why do we set limits in our lives? Why do so many people choose to live within their comfort zones?*

That same Friday night at 8:00, I headed out on a run. Yeah, I know what you're thinking: "Who runs on Friday nights?" Most people are either unwinding from the long week, partying with their friends, or hanging out with their families. I admit I don't normally run on Friday nights, either, but a sudden jolt of motivation pushed me out the door. I did not set a time goal or a distance goal; I just wanted to run *without limits*. Once I got going, I thought, "Ok, maybe I should just run all night."

What was going on? Why were these extreme thoughts entering my head?

No, I did not run all night. I ran for two hours, still a formidable outing for a Friday night.

That was the night the Limitless mindset really hit me. Too many times we create self-made barriers in our lives. We convince ourselves we cannot do something. We convince ourselves that we are not athletic enough or don't have the time. And then what happens? We end up cutting ourselves short on life-changing experiences. Maybe it's our society. Society is full of vulgarity, pessimism, and mediocrity. This negative culture beats us down. It wears on us. People fall into the trap of living an "average" existence because that is what society expects us to do.

"True human heartbreak is reaching your final moments and realizing that you wasted the most important gift that was given to you—the chance to present your magnificence to the world around you." This powerful quote is from Robin Sharma, author of *The Leader Who Had No Title*, a book I highly recommend.

I am always amazed how we allow negative self-talk to dictate our day-to-day lives. This negative perception becomes our reality. An equally negative mindset takes control of our beliefs and values, and we are doomed to mediocrity.

There are two ways to go: you either believe in yourself and take on challenges or you devalue yourself and adopt a cannot-do mindset. "I'm too fat." "I'm not tall enough." "I look horrible in this outfit." "I can't get to the gym today." "I can't eat healthy food." "I can't get a good job."

These daily thoughts alter our beliefs, our behaviors, and our way of life. They create limits on our true potential and barriers toward reaching our goals. Our beliefs are the product of thoughts and practices repeated over and over until they are cemented into our conscious minds as individual truths and reality. Pessimistic thinking will negatively influence our capability to achieve the goals and aspirations that we seek. I know from experience that when a decision has been made to embark on any goal, pessimistic thoughts will not and cannot support the journey. The more we can do to circumvent this type of thinking, the more optimistically we can live our lives. I try to make it a daily practice to limit, if not eliminate completely, the negative thoughts that enter my head on a regular basis. Conditioning the mind to do this takes work. I know because I work at it every day. It does not just happen overnight.

I have found that consistent, positive thinking and daily affirmations are needed to rebuild the internal thought process. I tell my students and my kids that the first step is to believe in yourself and make a practice of putting positive thoughts into your head. "I will get in the best shape of my life." "I will shop for and cook healthy foods." "I can do one more repetition." "I can go five more minutes on the treadmill." "I take responsibility for the things I want." "I will inspire my family today."

These are the kinds of thoughts that become real when you truly start believing in them.

Whether we are physically gifted or not, we all have the ability to improve our attitude. I am a big proponent of optimistic thinking and living. I am truly sold on the fact that your attitude affects your entire life, either positively or negatively. I also believe unequivocally that having the right attitude will change your life.

When we improve our attitude, limits are broken and the mind starts to believe that anything is possible.

Adjusting my attitude is the first step I take when facing a challenging task. I do everything in my power not to impose limits on myself. I try my best not give in to pessimistic people who criticize or condemn. I refuse to accept the status quo and eschew the term "average." Rough times are meant to provide motivation; I firmly believe this. We cannot get caught up in living a mediocre life. We all have the opportunity to accomplish the amazing, but it takes personal responsibility and accountability to make it happen.

Without really knowing it at the time, the Limitless philosophy was starting to formulate.

The next morning, I was on a bike ride with my good friend and training partner, Josh Hickey, and we began talking about this topic.

"Why do people set limits on themselves?" I asked.

"I think many people aspire for specific things, but aren't willing to push themselves to get there," he replied. "The limits they've imposed on themselves, either consciously or unconsciously, are stopping them from achieving what they want. People have a comfort zone and often set limits to stay comfortable."

When I first met Josh, I immediately saw his passion for life, and it was contagious.

Josh doesn't have special-endurance DNA on his side. He's worked his butt off to attain his current fitness level. Once he committed himself to his ultra-distance sport, he dove in head first and never looked back.

Something that strikes me about Josh is his constant push for improvement. Immediately after a race, he begins looking ahead for the next goal.

"Just enjoy this one, Josh," I tell him. But no, he is already devising a plan for his next race, his next challenge, his next adventure.

Josh has competed in and completed many major endurance events, including The Pine to Palm one-hundred-mile ultra-distance run in 2010 and multiple Ironman races. He does 50k training runs for "fun." Yeah, you read that right: for fun. This is a guy who always has a smile on his face and something positive to say.

When I bounced the Limitless idea off of him, I knew he would be crazy enough to join in and would be willing to help me in any way he could.

Before I officially announced the Limitless project to the community, I needed to start training. As I said earlier, I am not an "ultra-runner." I have built a solid base of triathlon fitness, but ultra-distance running was brand new for me. I needed to devise a plan. Step one: don't just talk about it. Step two: put together a training regimen. So Josh and I scheduled various self-supported ultra-distance marathons as part of our training plan. Step three: start running . . . lots!

The first planned run was a midnight-to-sunrise run. Sounds fun, right?

It actually sounded kind of nutty, but this would be the beginning of my ultra-distance lifestyle. This run would be my first taste of the ultra-distance world.

Let me be clear about one thing: you don't need to run long distances in the middle of the night to break down limits and barriers. This was my way; this was my individual challenge and endeavor. This was how I wanted to push myself mentally, physically, and spiritually. This was how I wanted to prove that anything is possible if you put in the effort.

Mark Twain once said, "If everyone was satisfied with themselves, there would be no heroes."

Finding ways to stay motivated and positively mold who we are as people will cement that "never stop" approach. That is why I am not a fan of "staying the same" or embracing the status quo. It is my personal value to always look for personal growth and forward movement. It is my way of creating enthusiasm toward living life fully every day.

We had an idea, and we put it into action. With this midnight-to-sunrise run, I was embarking on something entirely new and pushing my own physical and mental limits. I was excited but also a bit nervous. I definitely had some questions in my head leading up to this first ultra-run. First, how would my body hold up? Except for the marathon in the Ironman, I had never come close to running for six hours. This would by far be my longest run. Would it take an emotional toll on my body? Would I run into nagging issues like blisters, chafing, and pain? I had never experienced this "ultra-distance world," and I was about to enter the unknown.

CHAPTER 5

....

THE FIRST LIMIT BREAKER

The Midnight-to-Sunrise Run

Life still had to happen all day Friday despite our "plan."

Work started at 5:00 a.m., just like it did every day. I had a business to run. Clients needed to be trained. I stayed focused. These people deserved my very best. That's what they paid for, and they never received anything less from me or any of my trainers.

I made sure to eat and stay hydrated all morning. Friday is busy at CFA, and this particular Friday I had five training sessions throughout the morning. It's not like I could just sit around. Nor did I want to. When I train my clients, I am active and involved; that's what makes it fun.

Once my morning sessions were over, however, my afternoon and evening were fairly clear, so I made a point to rest and relax in preparation. Normally, I'm not a down-time person, but with a six-hour, midnight to 6:00 a.m. run staring me in the face, I forced myself to slow down.

Once 6:00 p.m. rolled around, I had an easily digestible meal of pasta and ground turkey. At 8:00, I rested my eyes for a couple hours. I was pretty excited for the adventure ahead, and I only managed about sixty minutes of solid sleep. Before I knew it, the clock chimed 11:00. I took a quick shower to wake up. I brewed coffee, ate a Cliff bar, and packed my gear for the night ahead.

I showed up at Josh Hickey's house a half hour later to the sight of a massive aide station stocked with drinks and snacks for our night ahead. Hickey was taking this experiment as seriously as I was, and I was grateful.

Nutrition for endurance sports is just as important as the actual training. Moreover, a nutrition plan for ultra-running is different than the nutrition plan I used for triathlons. I needed foods that would fuel my tank while at the same time not wreaking havoc on my stomach. This is easier said than done, and I found this out the hard way during the Ironman in Arizona. Throughout the bike portion, I consumed way too much of a sugary electrolyte drink that just ended up sitting in my stomach. When I transitioned from my bike into the run, my stomach was heavy, bloated, and in knots. My legs weren't a problem. They felt great, but the issues with my stomach stopped me from executing my run plan. At mile twelve, I hurried into a port-a-potty and made myself throw up. The result wasn't pretty, but it turned out to be the best thing I did that day. I immediately felt better. I found my stride again and ran strong for the entire second half of the marathon. Today I continue to explore the best nutrition plan for my body, knowing it's always a work in progress.

Josh and I headed out at 11:45 p.m. I wore a headlamp, a fuel belt around my waist, and headphones in my ears. My mindset couldn't have been better: I was ready to run all night. We took off running side by side, chitchatting about everything under the sun. Josh is a great running partner because we inevitably get into conversations that help time pass without getting too serious.

I know this much: running with a good friend is always better than running solo. If conversation happens, cool. If it's silent and we don't feel like talking, that's ok too. What's important is knowing someone else is out there going through similar emotions and physical duress. It's the power of empathy.

An hour into the run, we both zoned out. We opened our minds and got in tune with our bodies. I turned the volume on my music down low so I could listen to my thoughts and digest my emotions. That is most definitely another reason why I run; it is the perfect way to get in tune with my spirit and my soul, and with my body and my mind. Sometimes my thoughts rumble inside my head. Other times, the thoughts go silent and I slip into a state of meditation.

When all is said and done, that is what running is for me: a meditation. The distractions of life are gone. Negative stress releases. The focus is on my breathing, on each foot striking the earth, and on the person running next to me. It gives me a sense of good old-fashioned liberation, that sense of freedom that brings life into balance.

The plan was to break the run up into three twelve-mile segments so we could come back to our aide station, refuel, sit for a few minutes and recharge. Breaking the run up into three two-hour sessions made for a better outlook. Breaking down our goal made for a better mindset. As we neared the six-mile mark, we made our way to the outskirts of town, running parallel to the local Visalia airport. Both Hickey and I had run this route many times before, but never in the middle of night. It was dark and quiet at 1:00 a.m. in the morning. The only light came from our headlamps as they illuminated the road and a half moon in the sky that painted our path with a misty glow.

Surprisingly, time flew the first ten miles. We were running nine-minute miles, which is a good ultra-distance pace. We were three miles away from our first break, and it felt like we had only been running thirty minutes. We were off to a good start.

The temperature plunged along with the deepening night, and my hands and arms were freezing as we headed down the home stretch of our first leg. We finished the first loop in two hours. It was now 1:50 a.m. At our first break, I added an extra layer to keep my core warm and covered my arms with arm warmers. I ate half a Snickers bar, drank a few sips of a Mountain Dew, and refilled my bottle with half water and half Gatorade. I stretched briefly and was ready to head out on loop two.

We decided to take another route for the second interval. This route would lead us through the downtown streets of Visalia, which at 2:00 a.m. was pretty strange. The roads were essentially empty. The few people who were still out, probably from their late-night bar escapades, definitely gave us some weird looks. There we were, running gear on, headlamps shining bright, running through the streets at 2:30 in the morning. So, yeah, we probably deserved a weird look or two.

We hit the twenty-mile mark at around 3:00 a.m. This is where my mind really started to wander and the occasional body experience put a smile on my face. For the next hour, my mind was on cruise control. Looking back, I recall almost nothing about the miles we covered. I was just focused on putting one foot in front of the other.

When I got around to analyzing things, I realized I was still running strong. My body felt surprisingly good. It didn't feel like I had been running twenty-six miles. I was excited turning the corner to head back to our aide station for the second time. I was hungry, needed to refuel and stretch my legs, but I was definitely ready for the last push.

At one point I looked over at Josh and said, "We should try and hit forty miles." He looked at me as if Mr. Crazy had entered the room and he wasn't about to listen. So I told myself, *Just hit this last loop and we'll call it a night. Or a morning. Or whatever.*

I ate the other half of my Snickers bar, drank a few more sips of Mountain Dew, and had two Cliff shot blocks. The quick sugars were just enough to restore my energy.

We left for loop three at 4:00 a.m., my normal wake-up time. They talk about a "runner's high," and I think I had it right about then. Remember, this was my first taste of an ultra-distance run. Every feeling, every thought, every emotion was new to me. The last loop I did mostly by myself. Josh was not feeling 100 percent (he had been recovering from a cold) and only ran about five miles before calling it a night.

Running on your own in the dark—with no cars, no one to talk to, and barely able to see the ground in front of you—is eerie. My body was getting tired. My mind was definitely worn out. My music was starting to aggravate.

At 4:45 a.m., I turned off the music and allowed my mind to go where it would.

I had taken the same route that we had on our first loop, and by the time I reached the outskirts of town, my mind was in and out of the zone. I was running strong one minute and thinking about how tired I was the next. This ping-pong of emotion was a small but very significant taste of ultra-distance running.

I made it to the thirty-three mile mark. I stopped and walked for two minutes. I drank some fluids and took a moment to recharge my thoughts and give myself a pep talk for a strong finish.

I said, "It's just you and mother nature, Justin. Let's handle this and finish strong."

I set a strong eight-minute-per-mile pace, and it felt good. My running cadence became quick and explosive, my heart rate controlled. I wasn't breathing hard and settled into a good rhythm.

Endorphins are a powerful chemical, and they proved to be a great ally during this last stretch. I felt the best I had all night over the last three miles. As I came around the last few turns, I was completely in tune with my thoughts and my physicality.

"Limitless," I said aloud and turned the corner to Hickey's house.

I was done; thirty-six miles completed. It was 6:00 a.m., the sun was rising, and I could see the beautiful mountains lining the valley wall. I took it all in. This was my longest run yet, and it felt right. I logged in:

- Total distance: 36.1 miles
- Time: 5 hours 45 minutes
- Calories burned: 3861
- Calories consumed during: 1000 (166 calories/hour)
- Average pace: 9:33 min./mile

After some food that Josh had graciously prepared, I headed home. I took a hot shower, ate some more, and fell into a deep, dreamless sleep.

My midnight-to-sunrise adventure had come to an end, but the Limitless journey was just beginning. I was invigorated and motivated. Running these long distances gave me a new focus. These ultra-runs would challenge not only my physical prowess but also my mental, emotional, and spiritual self. I looked forward to that.

Every time I completed a long run, I learned something new, a lesson I would share with friends and family and try to incorporate into my client training.

I'd discovered one thing: breaking limits was exhilarating for me. I wanted more.

CHAPTER 6

....

CREATING LIMITLESS

The mission started to take shape.

It took a few brainstorming sessions with Hickey and a few more training runs, but an idea was formulating.

I discussed a plan for putting together an inspirational documentary with my brother Josh, a talented filmmaker, producer, and videographer, and it made sense that Limitless could be a part of it, if not at the very heart. We still didn't know the exact story line, but we did know we wanted to produce something that would motivate the masses, no small feat.

Josh had started his film career at the age of ten assisting our Uncle Dan, a filmmaker in his own right, on video shoots. Now Josh is a producer for Time Warner Media in Los Angeles. He has produced and directed numerous documentaries, short films, television commercials, and music videos. We are very close. Maybe it's the indefatigable determination and never-back-down attitude that we share. Growing up, we did everything together. Our fights were epic, but our dislike for each other (at least when the blows were landing) only lasted a few minutes. "Forget and forgive" came naturally to us, I suppose. I was the one who took Josh to his first high school party, and I was the one who gave him his first beer. He became a placekicker just like me. Of course, I was better than he was. And of course, he'd make the same claim. No matter.

These days, we share a great friendship. We are honest with each other and keep one another fully accountable. Sometimes this accountability issue leads to disagreements, but, just like when we were kids, we forgive each other and move on.

As the Limitless project began to coalesce in my head, I picked up the phone and threw my ideas at Josh to see how he'd react. One day I said, "Maybe I should just run to Los Angeles." A part of me was joking. Another part was dead serious.

"Dude, are you serious? That would be nuts," he replied with equal elements of sarcasm and surprise. Then he said, "Think you can do that?"

I said, "That's the whole point right there. Anything is possible, bro. When you believe in yourself and surround yourself with positive people, you start to develop an I-can mindset and it's all possible."

After that conversation, I bounced the idea off a few of the more accomplished ultra-runners in the area. With Hickey by my side, we started conversing about a number of extreme endurance ideas.

We first looked at running thirty miles a day for ten consecutive days. We nixed that idea out-of-hand because anything that took that long was unrealistic given such daily commitments as work and family and general life responsibilities.

Next we contemplated the idea of running fifty miles a day over six consecutive days. Did that fit the definition of "extreme endurance?"

"That's not tough enough," one of the guys I was consulting with said.

I had to chuckle. "Wait, fifty miles a day for six straight days is not tough enough? What the hell?"

Then I reminded myself that I was talking to guys who regularly ran fifty- and one-hundred-mile races throughout the year. In other words, these ultra-running events are nothing short of crazy. To really hit that insane level, we came to the conclusion that I needed to run at least sixty miles a day. The meeting broke up after settling on a proposal that called for running three hundred miles in four or five days.

As I drove home that night, I kept thinking, *What the hell am I getting myself into?* Here I was talking about running three hundred miles when I hadn't even run an organized marathon yet. Call me crazy. Call me extreme. But my motivation was high and this project was starting to sculpt itself.

The first step was to set a goal. Accountability does one thing: it forces the required action. And since I am an action taker, once I introduced the goal, preparation commenced. Once the project was formally announced, there would be no looking back. It was time to become an ultra-distance runner. I was fully committed. Now it was time to put together a blueprint for executing the project.

I will fully admit that moving into unfamiliar territory and pushing past my limits created some anxiety. I saw this as a positive. This was an ambitious goal, and I had no clue how my body would hold up. The unknowns of ultra-running scared me. The good news was that I have always believed in myself. With every goal, I have always created a positive consciousness and a mindset to succeed.

Failure is not an option in my mind; that's my mindset. The truth is, however, that creating this type of mindset takes work. And while such a forthright attitude has been a part of my life for a very long time, I still focus on it every day.

Yet, here I was entertaining the notion of running three hundred miles in four or five days. Crazy, to be sure. Yes, I was a bit naïve during the early stages of the Limitless project, but that naiveté probably worked to my advantage. I didn't know exactly what I was getting into, which, in many ways, kept the ball moving forward.

It is often said that ambition is a double-edged sword. If crazy ambition forces you to grow and expand your limits, it is also the source of major risks. Risk often leads to significant failure. But all of life is a gamble and living too carefully just puts you in an average place. Average is not in my DNA. If you're reading this, it's probably not in your DNA either.

We initially titled our expedition the "Valley-to-Valley 300-Mile Run." The name made sense since we would be running from the Central Valley into the San Fernando Valley. We used MapMyRun.com to study the various routes available to us, and I eventually penciled out a course that looked like this:

- Depart from Visalia;
- Run to the small rural cities of Exeter and Porterville;
- Make our way into Bakersfield;
- Run into the Mojave Desert;
- Climb into the Angeles National Forest;
- Run into Los Angeles;
- Finish at the Santa Monica Pier.

Looking at the map, most of the running would be done on country roads or "run accessible" highways. The only part of the route that I was not quite sure about was the city running once we arrived in Los Angeles. Tricky. Very tricky. But instead of sweating it, I decided we would just have to handle that once we got there.

I officially announced the project on my Facebook page in late March 2012 with this statement:

My new journey begins . .

Limitless: *Valley-to-Valley 300-mile run.*

LIMITLESS

What does Limitless mean to you? To me, Limitless is eliminating self-made barriers that stagnate optimal living. Can you or can't you? I want to inspire people to challenge themselves to live with an "I can" mindset. Life is what you make it, and I truly believe that optimistic living enables people to achieve their goals and reach success.

My name is Justin Levine. I am an inspired fitness and triathlon coach and endurance athlete who is on a mission to motivate and encourage this mindset. I am putting together a project called the "Valley-to-Valley 300-Mile Run." This ultra-distance run will start in my hometown of Visalia and take me through the heart of the Central Valley. I will make my way down into Southern California with a planned finish at the Santa Monica Pier.

My goal: four days to complete, which equates to seventy-five miles per day.

Limitless goes well beyond physical elements. It taps into the mental and spiritual sides of living life. When limits are broken, life can be truly cherished. Physical achievements can be accomplished. Relationships can be built. "Impossible" becomes realistic.

My planned departure date is October 16 at 8:00 a.m. Stay tuned for updates and information regarding this epic journey.

Once this post was made on my Facebook page, Limitless . . . became . . . real.

The next step was announcing the project throughout the community. I wanted others to get involved and be familiar with the mission. I knew that the more people who got involved, the greater the impact would be.

At first, many people didn't truly understand why or what I was doing.

"You're doing what?" they would ask. "That's seems a bit extreme."

Messages like these were the norm in the beginning. The true significance of Limitless didn't really make its influence until later in the year, as the run grew closer.

I do remember one specific Facebook comment, however, that proved particularly motivating. It read:

This is running, not cycling. The physical stresses on the body are huge and the caloric/hydration needs can be prohibitive, especially in four days. I have a feeling it will take eight to ten days covering forty or so miles a day. Each day will also become progressively more difficult.

I laughed when I read this post, though there was an element of truth in the writer's words: this was an insane proposition. Instead of his words sparking insecurities or doubts, however, I found motivation and drive in them and used them over the coming months to keep me inspired and focused.

I announced the project to the long-standing Visalia Runners Club. They invited me to their club meeting, and I'm not quite sure if everyone in attendance that night conceptualized my announcement. It seemed so informal. I said:

Thank you for having me here tonight. I just wanted to let everyone know of a project I am putting together called the Valley-to-Valley Run. *I will be running three hundred miles in four days, starting in Visalia and finishing at the Santa Monica Pier. I will make the run in four days to prove that anything is possible, that limits can be broken, and that life can be lived at high levels. If you would like to get involved, please let me know. We are looking for pace runners and assistance with the project.*

The room went awkwardly silent.

"Does anyone have questions?" I asked. There were no questions.

The club president reclaimed the microphone and said, "Thanks for joining the meeting, Justin. We look forward to hearing more about the run. See you soon."

It wasn't a complete loss. The club president also gave me permission to announce the project at the local half-marathon race schedule for the coming weekend.

When the time came, Michael Baumann, a good friend and member of the Visalia Runners Club, read the short and sweet announcement at the post-race expo. The announcement said:

"Justin Levine, a well-respected member of the Visalia fitness community, will be running three hundred miles in four days to prove, as he puts it, that anything is possible. He will start in Visalia and run to Santa Monica. He hopes to spread the Limitless life message and inspire others to break their own individual limitations. If you would like to get involved, contact Justin for more information."

It was another awkward announcement. You could barely hear his words due to the hustle and bustle of the expo. The statement was monotone and dry, and you could tell Michael was reading off a sheet of paper. Most people heard "three-hundred-mile run in four days" and some heard "Visalia to Santa Monica," but not much else.

It wasn't a complete loss. A few people came up to me with questions. I hopefully had the answers, but I too was walking on unfamiliar ground.

Nonetheless, we had used the two forums to achieve our goal of announcing the project to the community. Small steps. I wasn't disappointed by the response. We wanted to get the ball rolling, and we had done that.

One positive was the interest taken in the project by my good friend Jim Barnes. Jim had attended the meeting at the Visalia Runners Club where I first announced the project, and he was intrigued with the idea. He called me later that night asking for more details. He wanted to make sure that he had heard me correctly.

"Did you say three hundred miles in four days? Was that correct?" he asked.

"Crazy, but true," I said.

"I like crazy. How can I get involved?" Jim asked.

"Well, I'd love any help you can give."

"How are you planning to carry your food and water? Have you given any thought to that?" he asked.

"I have to admit that we haven't," I told him. "Any ideas?"

"Well, I wouldn't be much use to you as a pace runner. Not at my age. But I could bike and be there for support."

This was a great idea, and we talked more about it. We decided that having a cyclist by our side throughout the run would help tremendously with fluid and food distribution. This was not an easy job, however. Not just anyone could do it. We needed somebody who had extensive knowledge of endurance sports. That was Jim. He was not only familiar with endurance sports, but, at sixty-seven years old and a retired schoolteacher, he had long been into fitness and community service. His philanthropic work had served thousands of people in the community over the years. He began competing in endurance sports in the 80s, running marathons and triathlons back when these sports were in their infancy.

Jim was responsible for putting together Triathlon Across America to raise money for the Jeff Barnes Brain Injury Foundation. This nonprofit organization provides assistance to brain-injured individuals and their families through advocacy, resources, and financial assistance. Jim would swim, bike, and run at races throughout the country, raising awareness for his foundation. His philanthropy is truly amazing. He has worked with Team in Training (TNT), Police Activities League (PAL), the Visalia Rescue Mission, Students International, and many others.

Jim's phone call could not have been timelier. The skills and knowledge he brought to the table for the Limitless project were destined to be an integral component as we moved forward. He was the perfect man for the job, and I could not have been more grateful.

Following our initial announcements, we knew we needed to do a better job communicating with the community in general and the fitness community in particular about the project, so my brother Josh created a website depicting the Limitless philosophy. This outlet helped define our project and opened the door for people to ask questions or share their comments.

We also created a Facebook page to help spread the message, and the "likes" began pouring in. The plan was to use the page to promote positive posts, give our followers training updates, and share sponsorship news. It was a great avenue to communicate with people interested in our project.

The next step in the process was to form a committee of positive people to build and promote the Limitless project. I couldn't do this by myself. When we put the word out, the response was unbelievable. We had community leaders, local runners, friends, and family step up to the plate and join our efforts. The committee planned to meet once a month beginning in April 2012. As soon as we started planning in earnest, the event grew by leaps and bounds. This was no longer just about some guy running three hundred miles in four days. Suddenly we were spearheading a massive project to create optimism throughout the community. Let me rephrase that: "Throughout the world."

The goal was to bring together a group of motivating and optimistic individuals to build the Limitless platform, people who related to our message and wanted to deliver it to the world.

What we found was an audience far more responsive than I ever anticipated. It's simple, really. Everyone has limits. And the idea of "some guy" running three hundred miles in four days did more than just intrigue people; it also motivated them to battle their own limitations.

There was so much to talk about with the committee during the first few meetings: sponsorships, fundraising strategies, route logistics, pace runners, brochures, marketing for the event, and the overall production of the movie. It seemed that once the seed was planted, everyone on the committee became inspired and really wanted to build upon the momentum we had and spread the word. I was humbled. What seemed like a simple idea was turning into a colossal, extremely important expedition. Suddenly, the "Valley-to-Valley" title did not fit the nature of the project, and we wanted a name that gave a better description of our platform. We settled on LIMITLESS—Life in Motion. We also modified our four-day timeframe to one hundred hours. We figured this would give us an extra morning to reach our destination.

So it became LIMITLESS—Life in Motion—a 300-Mile Run in 100 Hours.

I was embarking on my own Limitless journey to prove to people that life is what you make it, that our self-imposed limits can be surpassed, that pushing our boundaries can and will lead to optimal living, and that *anything is truly possible.*

This became our platform, and we wanted to share the message with as many people as possible. We also set a goal of raising $20,000 for the Central Valley Team in Training (TNT) chapter. TNT fundraises for the Leukemia and Lymphoma Foundation. We chose this organization because they are very connected to the endurance lifestyle. The work these people do to raise money is nothing short of remarkable. In over twenty-five years as an organization, they have trained more than 600,000 participants to complete a half or full marathon, cycling or triathlon event, or hiking adventure, and have raised over $1.4 billion to help with blood cancer research and treatment.

I have personally built strong relationships with members of the local Team in Training group in Visalia over the years. I lend my support by giving nutrition and training workshops through-out the year, and their support for the Limitless concept and our platform made for a perfect fit.

CHAPTER 7

....

YOU GET KNOCKED DOWN, YOU GET BACK UP

There is a saying: *The greatest glory is not in never falling, but in rising every time we fall.*

It's mesmerizing to think what three hundred miles of running looks like. I computed the approximate number of footsteps one would take over such an unprecedented distance. An ultra-runner takes approximately eight-five foot strikes per minute (counting one foot), which equates to approximately 765 steps per mile. Translated, that means someone running three hundred miles will take in the area of 229,500 steps! That is equivalent to running 11.5 marathons. It's like running 1,200 laps around a four-hundred-yard track.

Here is another calculation I couldn't resist making. A 140-pound man running at a speed of 5.5 mph burns between 600-800 calories per hour (depending on the terrain, speed, and individual). So if my goal was to run fifteen to seventeen hours per day, I would burn between 9,000 and 13,600 calories each day! Multiply that by four days and you get 36,000 to 54,400 calories gone! Yeah, I am hungry just thinking about that.

Part of the planning process, therefore, was dealing with this extraordinary problem. During my training runs, I practiced nutritional strategies and found some remedies that worked and some that didn't. Nutrition is different for these ultra-distance runs. When you run longer distances at a slower pace, food is absorbed and digested differently. I learned this during my training and put it in my memory bank as the longer days approached.

Fighting through physical fatigue was another inevitable aspect of the endeavor we were planning. My body would go through tremendous stress and anguish, but the mental and emotional fatigue was something of an unknown, something almost mysterious, and something I knew would take extreme determination to push through.

Some say that ultra-running is more of a spiritual event than an athletic event. Dean Karnazes, an advocate of this viewpoint, put it this way: "If you want to run, run a mile; if you want a different life, run a marathon; but if you want to talk to God, run an ultra."

Once the body hits its limits, the mind takes over. Once the mind starts to weaken and begins playing tricks on you, it is up to the spirit to carry on. That "spiritual determination" needed to become a very strong part of my makeup to help me overcome the pain my body would be experiencing.

Ultra-runner Marshall Ulrich, one of the legends of the sport, talks about his experiences on pain, suffering, and endurance, saying:

"I've always seen endurance as a means to an end, a way of squeezing every last ounce out of life, a way to see more, experience more, accomplish more, live more. So, yes, I've been willing to deal with discomfort for long periods of time—spending hours squeezing through caves so tight they felt suffocating . . . .

"Perseverance is about scoring a victory over the difficulty, pain, or discomfort that you choose to endure for the sake of your sport and the personal rewards you get out of it. But you can't 'attack' suffering as if it were your competitor; to win this one, you have to accept it. This means recognizing that you made a choice, swallowing your complaints, and finding a higher purpose for what you're doing. It requires that you transcend the physical, have confidence that you'll succeed, know that there will be an end, and take quitting off the table. In doing all this, you prove to yourself that the only limits are in your mind. You discover what you're made of. It's more than you think, no matter your past, your genetics, your gender, or your age."

For me, the run was a metaphor for life. When I get knocked down, I simply get back up. When I'm tired, I rest. I put one foot in front of the other. I find motivation. At times, I "run" hard. At times, I pace myself. I'm consistent no matter what. I find others to inspire. I find others to inspire me.

The run was my personal challenge, even as it was a challenge so many others had chosen to join. For me, stretching one's personal limits means getting uncomfortable. Feeling uncomfortable means you're growing, changing, challenging. Deep down, I believe life is what you make it. Waking up each day ready to squeeze every ounce of your potential is, to my way of thinking, the only way to go.

I want people to live with strong health, proper nutrition, personal improvement, and a daily mindset to be happy. I want people to focus on the positives. I want people to test their limits. I say go for the ultimate! Those are words I live by. Those are words I infuse into my personal training. I want my kids to think that way. I want my employees to think that way. I wanted my Limitless team to think that way.

We all know people who go through each day of their lives with a pessimistic view of the world. We all know people who focus on the negatives. "Can't" is a word too many people use. "Just getting through the day" is a motto too many people employ. I know that "self-belief" is not a part of everyone's vocabulary. I know there are a lot of people who wake up unhappy. They're good with the status quo. They're good with staying comfortable.

I fight this type of mindset at every turn because I fear it will adversely affect my physical, mental, and spiritual health. You may know the feeling. I, for one, can't have that. My passion—which is more like my religion—is to live my life with optimism, belief, determination, and discipline. I have experienced how this outlook positively affects my physical, mental, and spiritual health, and that is enough to keep me motivated.

We all seek to inspire. This passion for life is, I suppose, my way of inspiring people to be more than they ever thought they could be. Likewise, we all seek to motivate. And this positive outlook is, I suppose, my way of motivating others in the belief that that life can be lived at high levels.

This ultra-run was real. It was planned. The date was set. The public knew about it. I was embarking on the most daunting challenge I had ever undertaken. I was preparing my mind, body, and soul for this life-altering experience, and there was no looking back.

CHAPTER 8

....

TRAINING, RUNNING, AND LIFE

Warren Buffet likes to say: "The most important ingredient to success is obsession."

Well, he certainly describes me to a T. When I set a goal, I freely admit that I become obsessed with achieving it. Just ask my wife, kids, family, or friends. Even my business associates have had a taste of my bull-dog, never-quit-until-you-get-there mentality.

To me, obsession is not a bad thing, especially when it is directed toward positive ends and the prospect of doing good. I always do my best to find a balance with the many important aspects of my busy life, but when you've set a goal that 100 percent of the people you talk to describe as outrageous—like running three hundred miles in one hundred hours—some important things are bound to be shortchanged, if not sacrificed. My family time, my social life, my friendships: all took a back seat as I trained for Limitless. Stephanie and I had an eighteen-mouth-old daughter at the time and missing Olivia JoJo even for a day was painful; I did my best to minimize this. I watched less TV and spent less time socializing outside the home so that I could spend my limited free time with family.

The exceptions were my businesses. They represented my livelihood; that's how I support my family. So the long hours spent running my businesses and working with my clients would remain a constant even as I trained. No shortcuts there.

I am quite rigid when it comes to time management, and that didn't change as I started my Limitless training. My daily schedule looks like this: go to work early, take a midday break, and then work through the afternoon and very often into the evening. We never cancel client appointments, emergencies excepted. And even in the case of emergencies, my staff and I always try to cover for one another. My training, therefore, had to fit into an already busy schedule. I didn't complain. I was lucky to have a great team around me and a personal dedication to using every free moment available to me.

Part of effective time management is taking care of life's priorities. If I don't have a firm hold on my schedule, chaos is the byproduct, and the byproduct of chaos is time wasted.

Sometime during the day on Sunday, I spend forty-five to sixty minutes arranging my week ahead. I start with my business appointments; I add in my client training sessions. I have another section for general business tasks. I make time for reading and writing. I make a point of highlighting family time with Stephanie and Olivia (and these days with Bobbi Jo, our newest addition). I schedule naps, meals, my own training and workouts, and anything else that is needed for what I describe as a "successful week."

If it's important, it gets scheduled. This has always been my mantra regarding time management.

During this Sunday planning time, I also write out all my "to dos" for the week. Once Monday begins, one by one, I start taking care of these responsibilities. Once I finish a task, a fluorescent highlight goes through the finished assignment. This gives me a sense of victory. At the end of the week, when I have all my completed tasks neatly highlighted, I feel a major wave of confidence and self-esteem. I've had a successful and productive week.

Personal improvement happened. I wasn't just sitting there keeping busy. I made things happen. I got closer to my goals. Multiply these ten to fifteen small weekly victories over a fifty-two-week year and I have something like 520 to 780 accomplished tasks. With the accumulations of all these small victories comes major achievement in so many areas.

Most high-level businesspeople create their own luck by demonstrating a potent and powerful work ethic. While I am nowhere close to my true potential, I am always striving for things like better time management, personal productivity, and life improvement. As these areas develop, I am able to have more freedom to be with my family, spend more quality time training, and, hopefully, grow closer to the life I envision for myself and my loved ones.

I am sure it is no surprise that running became a priority leading up to Limitless. I came into 2012 as a fair-to-midland triathlete with seven years of consistent triathlon training under my belt. I was not, however, an ultra-distance runner. My running schedule in preparation for the event called for sixty to one-hundred mile weeks. I am a big advocate of quality versus quantity in most anything I pursue, but I knew my running volume needed to increase in order to best prepare for this outrageous ultra-run.

Most of my running miles were slow and aerobic in nature. Speed was not a priority. I needed to be able to last and have stamina. It wasn't about running three hundred miles "fast."

I also incorporated swimming, biking, strength training, and mobility work into my training regimen. Swimming was a great way to build fitness without all the pounding on the body. Biking gave me a chance to get off my legs but also to have a two- to four- hour aerobic workout. Strength training was a component that tremendously assisted with injury prevention.

Running puts stress on the body. As a coach, I am always advising runners to add other elements to their program. They shouldn't just run and forget about these other components. Mobility is just as important as the running. Poor movement qualities are a precursor to injury. Tight ankles, immobile hips, and poor muscle flexibility doom the runner to chronic pain. I spend at least ten minutes every day working on my active mobility. As opposed to yoga or static stretching, I move. I perform dynamic drills meant to keep my body limber and mobile. Swimming, biking, strength training, and mobility drills were all components meant to aide in my running training. I was of the mind that becoming a complete athlete could only have positive and consistent ramifications on my running lifestyle, and I was seeing the results day by day.

If you are into sports of any kind, you know that injuries bring inconsistency into your training, and inconsistency is almost certain to impede your progress.

While running was my main focus, I knew that creating a balanced program would limit my chances of injury.

My typical training week leading up to Limitless looked like this:

- Monday—One hour steady run on treadmill (five to seven miles).
- Tuesday—Workout #1: one hour steady run with training partners (seven to nine miles); Workout #2: mobility and movement work to stay mobile and functional.
- Wednesday—Workout #1: one hour indoor bike with Tri Club; Workout #2: strength training/core work.
- Thursday—Workout #1: one hour tempo run (six to eight miles); Workout #2: swim with Tri Club.
- Friday—Off or one- to two-hour hour steady run if I needed to add volume to the week.
- Saturday—Long run of eighteen to thirty-five miles.

• Sunday—One- to two-hour run (six to twenty miles) or two-hour bike ride if I needed to get off my legs.

I had a distinct advantage: I love to train. Rarely does the thought of pressing the snooze button and sleeping an extra half-hour enter my mind. Ninety-nine percent of the time I get up, wash my face, eat a banana, and go out and complete my training.

It should be said, however, that I listen to my body. When I am physically and mentally drained, I skip that day's training or trade in my usual routine for something light. I encourage my clients to do the same and I would you as well.

Once I entered my 30s, I noticed a change in the way my body adapted to training. My recovery was just not as quick. I realized that I couldn't just push hard all the time. When I did, it inevitably led to overtraining, burnout, and ultimately injury. So I learned. Over the years, I have done pretty well at staying away from chronic injury (knock on wood). And if some type of pain or injury does arise, I handle the problem with proper rehabilitation and allow myself sufficient time to get back on my feet.

For me, constant management of my overall fitness program is a critical aspect to my long-term development. I am not just running to get fit. I want to be fit to run, to handle stress, and to have the energy to do all the things I want to do. I want to be fit so I can live life as fully as possible. This is a message my trainers and I share with our clients at the gym. It just makes sense.

Even though running was my main focus at the time, I always added in other modalities to keep my body strong, athletic, and durable. I always considered myself an athlete, and there were few sports I wouldn't try.

I came into my endurance lifestyle a strong athlete. I started weight training when I was eighteen. I loved it. My short stature was a plus; it enabled me to add muscle quickly. I used old-school body-building routines to grow muscle. However, once my focus turned to a triathlon and endurance lifestyle, heavy weight training was no longer a priority, nor was it an appropriate balance for the amount of running and biking I was doing. I turned my attention instead to functional strength routines.

Since I began training for endurance sports, I lost nearly twenty-five pounds. This was significant at the time, given my small frame.

As the year progressed and I was getting physically prepared, my confidence increased exponentially. I was starting to think that I could do this; the Limitless run was no longer a pipe dream, but a growing reality. I had days in my week where I would run to work, run to meetings, basically run everywhere I needed to go. It added miles to my week, and it prepared me for running multiple times during the course of a day. There would be a lot of stopping and starting over the one hundred hours that would go into running three hundred miles. Even the most prepared athletes run into daunting situations in ultra-running. Blisters, chaffing, and joint pain can stop a runner in his or her tracks. Hallucinations, mind games, and delirium are a few of the issues known to arise over the course of long run. Physical anguish is a given. You know that going in. What you also have to be prepared for are the mental and spiritual battles, the noise inside your head.

With each training run, I was learning more and more about these unique situations and how to handle them.

I had built my endurance to a point where running twenty-five miles was just a normal training day. Imagine that. In the months leading up to Limitless, I began running the equivalent of a marathon every Saturday or Sunday; all of a sudden I was looking at that as normal preparation. Some weekends my running mileage would exceed fifty miles over the two days. My body gradually adapted. I knew that I needed to complete numerous long runs to teach my body, as I liked to put it, "to go long."

In the weeks leading up to the run, I also knew I needed to up my training mileage during the workweek. When I wasn't working or spending time with my wife and daughter, I was running. I could have found resistance on the home front, but it was just the opposite. Stephanie and Olivia were in my corner all the way (or at least as much as an eighteen-month old can be). Stephanie understood what I was striving to achieve, and she was all in. I couldn't have done it without her.

In the months before Limitless, I completed any number of self-supported ultra-runs and heavy mileage weeks, and here is a sampling:

- March: Midnight to 6:00 a.m. Visalia run, thirty-six miles
- April: Visalia to Earlimart—thirty-three miles. Mid-month, we were leaving on a family vacation. That morning I was wondering how I could get a training session in before we left, so I packed our car the night before. That way Stephanie would only have to pack up Olivia and her things before we set off. I left several hours before she did and started running. This was a particularly boring run through the less-than-scenic Tulare County, so I listened to the audio version of *The Alchemist* in hopes of keeping my mind occupied.

It was 8:30 in the morning when Stephanie pulled the truck up next to me. What a sight for sore eyes. I took the earbuds out of my ears, jumped in the car, and our vacation officially started!

- April: "Vacation" training camp run—twenty-six-mile training run, 103-mile training week. After the Visalia-to-Earlimart run, we made our way to Washington to visit Stephanie's grandparents. I made this a vacation training camp. I would run every day. On our third day of vacation, I left Grandma's house and make my way south toward Seattle.

Once again, the plan was for Stephanie to pick me up enroute. I put in a good marathon-plus before Stephanie and our daughter caught up to me, and we drove the rest of the way to Seattle and enjoyed a terrific one-day visit.

• June: Visalia to Three Rivers, thirty-eight miles. I made this training run with Josh Hickey. We set out from my house and ran up and around the lake and into the surrounding mountains. I'd made this trek many times on my bike, and the views of the lake and the mountains were outstanding.

We met some other friends at mile sixteen and they joined us. I started feeling particularly strong at mile twenty and ran the last fifteen miles with an unexpected but rewarding ease. My fitness was at a high level and growing daily.

• July: Pacific Valley Training Camp—forty-mile run with four thousand feet of climbing, 110-mile training week. Each year, we take a camping trip with Stephanie's side of the family. It's always special and a trip I always look forward to. This year, I used the trip as a training camp with all the perks: high elevation, scenic running roads and challenging trails, and lots of rest and recovery.

Here's how it worked. Stephanie's mom and dad live forty miles south of the campground we were using. I would take off early in the morning from her parents' home with plenty of water and sufficient food and "meet" them at the campsite. My good friend Steve Juarez rode his bike next to me for this run. "Epic!" There is no other way to describe it with all the elevation gains, the miles we were covering, and the extraordinary terrain. I remember turning the last corner and seeing our campsite. A sight for sore eyes it was. I was elated.

A cold beer tasted good that day.

• July: twenty-five-mile run along the High Sierra Trail, five thousand feet of elevation and unsurpassed scenery!

• August: Exeter, California water tower to Lemon Cove, California and back, twenty-six miles.

- August: Exeter, California water tower to the Oak Tree and back, twenty-six miles.
- September: Arroyo Grande, three-day training camp—first day, forty-eight miles; second day, forty miles; third day, twenty-seven miles—115 miles total.

As you can see, there is no easy way to build endurance. You put in the time or it doesn't happen. Was I a nuisance to my family? At times, for sure. But I wanted them with me as often as possible so we could spend time together. Did I sacrifice time away from my family and ask them to sacrifice in return? Absolutely. These long runs could take upwards of six hours. By the time I would get home, I needed to recover. But I was fortunate. As I said, Stephanie understood what I was trying to achieve. I wanted her and Olivia to be proud of me; I kept them posted on everything I was doing and why. If I had to kick my feet up for a while and relax, they rarely complained. Limitless had become our mutual goal.

CHAPTER 9

....

DRESS REHEARSAL

We planned a training camp seven weeks before Limitless. This would give us a chance to see how our bodies would respond to running three consecutive days in a row. My brother would also be shooting footage for the documentary and observing the ins and outs of ultra-running firsthand.

We were lucky. My Aunt Chris and Uncle Robert allowed us to set up our training camp at their amazing home in Arroyo Grande. It was perfect for our needs. Maybe a little too perfect: we had a beautiful home to stay in and great food at every meal. Spoiled? Maybe just a little.

We researched the area and decided on three different point-to-point routes. Stephanie agreed to pick us up at each of our final destinations. The initial goal was to run forty-five miles the first day, forty miles the second day, and a marathon the third day. I was confident. My training had been going very well, and my body and mind felt strong. I also understood that a back-to-back training camp was going to push both our bodies and our minds. Moreover, this was the first time I would be running forty-plus miles in a single outing.

There was no perfect training strategy in preparation for a run of three hundred miles over one hundred hours. This was a work in progress. I was learning on the fly. Basically, I got out there and ran as much as I could and did my best to not get injured. One thing I did know: there was no shortcut. The key component was consistent hard work. One workout in and of itself was not important; it was the string of workouts consistently completed over the long haul that truly mattered.

Jim, Hickey, and I set out that first morning at 6:00 a.m., Jim on his bike, and Josh and I in our running gear. The plan was to run from Arroyo Grande to Lompoc over forty-five miles of moderately undulating terrain.

I can state one thing categorically. Running anything longer than a marathon is grueling, to say the least. There isn't an easy approach to this distance. It's literally putting one foot in front of the other, keeping up with nutrition, and grinding away.

We made our way out of town through the outskirts of Arroyo Grande, running through Nipomo, and eventually hitting the Cabrillo Highway/Highway 1. Most people envision Highway 1 running right along the coastline—which a good amount of it does—but the portion we were on at the time was inland.

We hit the eighteen-mile mark with relative ease and took a short break in the small Hispanic community of Guadalupe. We definitely got some odd looks, and why not. Here it was a Friday morning and three "gringos" were running (or riding, in Jim's case) through the town like it was the most natural thing in the world.

We stopped to refuel and get a quick bite to eat. Our spirits were high, and we continued through the city. Our ultra-running pace hovered around 9:45 minutes per mile. This was a comfortable and manageable pace that we could sustain for long periods. Shutting down the mind was more or less a necessity during a run of this length, but ours was not a trio given to silence. If it wasn't Josh talking about training or some type of nutritional element, it was Jim telling us stories meant to help time go by; the good news was that Jim was a better-than-average storyteller, and Josh and I were a captive audience.

Once we made it to the outskirts of Guadalupe, we needed to put our heads down and put some miles behind us. We fell into a pleasant and much-needed silence at this point. I shut my mind down and meditated. For me, just being quiet is one of the perks of ultra-running.

We veered off the Cabrillo Highway and began running on the barren roads of the Central Coast. The sun started to peek through the overcast coastal clouds. It wasn't necessarily hot, but the sun added another element to the equation. At the marathon mark, we started to hit long stretches of desolate road. We had not seen a town, roadside market, or gas station since our stop in Guadalupe, nearly fourteen miles back. Our water supply started to run low. That had us worried. Dehydration is a killer no matter what form of exercise you're participating in and even more so for long distance running.

Then we spotted a sign that read: *Cold drinks—two miles ahead.*

Jim took off on his bike and hurried down the road, only to find a boarded-up storefront and no running water. Not good. Especially since there were no other stores in town. Undaunted, Jim turned to plan B, which meant asking a local farmer if he could fill up our water bottles. Mission accomplished.

He returned with water to spare—though you really never have water to spare—and a fun story to tell.

The next ten miles took us in and around undulating hills. The weather was bone dry and the running was quiet and concentrated. We were going through water fast.

It was over this stretch that Josh felt the onset of dehydration. He adjusted his pace and fell behind slightly. He encouraged me to keep my pace up since I was running comfortably. We eventually arrived at the historic Vandenberg Air Force Base and made the swing back to Highway 1. We were eight miles from Lompoc, and the end was in sight.

Honestly, I couldn't believe how strong I felt at mile forty-three. I heard myself saying, "Hey, this ultra-stuff isn't that bad." (Yeah, right, just wait till later . . .)

With about four miles to go, Jim went back to ride the final miles with Josh, while I pushed on to the finish, running strong and feeling good.

A rush of endorphins and energy hit me as I turned into the parking lot where Stephanie was meeting us. I came in smiling, and she said, "I'm amazed at how fresh you look. How do you feel?"

"Way better than expected," I told her. We had run forty-eight miles in eight hours and forty-five minutes, the longest I had ever run. "The crazy thing is, I felt pretty darn strong the entire time."

"Congratulations," she said as Jim and Josh pulled into the lot, only a few minutes behind me. "You guys must be starving."

We were not only hungry, but thirsty and desperate to get off our feet. That night Josh and I soaked our legs in ice water, ate a hearty dinner, drank copious amounts of fluids, and went to bed early.

Another day of running was coming.

I woke up, got out of bed, and was struck by a singular thought: *Okay, my legs aren't too sore.*

You would think running forty-eight miles the day before would have created delayed muscle soreness. Eating quality food, cold-therapy sessions, and a light stretching routine definitely assisted the recovery process.

As an athlete, the recovery process is just as important as the training process. If you don't allow the body to recover and adapt to the stress applied in between training sessions, you then become that much more susceptible to injury and overtraining.

I am constantly pushing my body. That means asking the question, "Am I training smart?"

Training smart does not necessarily translate into training hard. I train hard but I also give tremendous attention to progression, nutrition, and recovery. I am in constant assessment of my body, continually looking for symptoms of overtraining. Interrupted or inconsistent sleep, nagging injuries, lack of performance, daily fatigue (even after a solid night's rest), decrease in appetite, lack of motivation, and persistent muscle soreness are just a few symptoms of overtraining. If any of these symptoms surface, I have disciplined myself to take as many as three days off or to implement what I call "light training days." In any case, I always schedule rest and recovery days into my regimen. Active recovery sessions keep the body sharp and strong and that, after all, is the goal of training in the first place.

The moment I woke up, I began drinking fluids. Dehydration hinders endurance athletes as much as any other problem, and combining three days of running back-to-back increases the chances of falling prey to this very dangerous issue. Hydration is always a priority. In fact, it is a lifestyle habit. I bring my water bottle everywhere I go.

Josh, Jim, and I ate breakfast, drank coffee, used the foam roller to loosen up our muscles, and did a dynamic warm-up to prepare for the upcoming day. Jim said a short prayer, reminding us to be thankful for the brotherhood and the ability to be physically active. He did this every morning. Jim was our spiritual mentor and his fellowship would be essential during our Limitless run.

We once again took off from my aunt and uncle's house. Today's goal was Montana de Oro State Park, a forty-mile trek. We headed west toward Pismo Beach, a small beach town located six miles from Arroyo Grande. We took a scenic three-mile route and made our way along the beach into Pismo. Not surprisingly, Jim didn't like this idea. Riding a bike on the sand hardly struck his fancy. Hickey and I, on the other hand, loved it. The sky was overcast, the waves were crashing not twenty feet away, and the surroundings were perfect. There is something so peaceful about running on the beach. It never ceases to move me. With the kinetic energy of the water and the music of the crashing waves, it's meditative and inspiring all at the same time.

We met our good friends Mark and Carol Richards at the ten-mile mark in Shell Beach. They would run a ten-mile stretch with us through the quaint little town of Avila Beach. The plan was then to take a fire road from Avila to Montana de Oro; MapMyRun.com showed a "through" road that looked accessible, but a security guard monitoring access quickly dashed our hopes of that route.

Thinking on our feet—no pun intended—we turned around and made our way to San Luis Obispo (SLO). Nothing wrong with a little detour, right?

Once there, we met up with Stephanie, eighteen-month-old JoJo (the joy of my life), and my brother's girlfriend, Robin. It is always good to see fresh and positive faces on runs as long as this one. It did wonders for my spirits.

We took a short break, which gave me time to hug my daughter. With the sun rising higher in the sky, we applied sunscreen in liberal doses. We ate a snack and replenished our water bottles. It was time for the next leg of our journey.

We took off on Los Osos Valley Road, a long, straight stretch that measured thirteen miles. It was during this stretch that I experienced my first down points of the weekend. My body was on the verge of rebelling, so I tilted my hat low on my head, put my eyes down, and tried my best to just zone out. Just keep those legs moving.

The next two hours were a rollercoaster of high and low energy points that seemed to come and go for no reason. Eventually, our pace stabilized around the ten-minute-per-mile mark. If we needed to eat something or felt the urge to slow our pace, we might slow to a fast walk for a short stretch, but we continued to march on. I felt my energy levels stabilize.

When we hit the seventy-five-mile mark for the two days we'd been running, I experienced a new "runner's high."

With eight miles to go, I felt very strong. As we made our way through the small towns of Baywood and Los Osos, my legs began to turn over a little faster and my running speed increased. "The horse smelled the barn," as the saying goes. The final half-mile was a steep climb that offered one last challenge. I pushed myself, knowing the end was near, and knowing we were on the verge of a new milestone.

It was all worth it when we made it to the summit. The view was nothing short of magnificent. The sun was out, the weather was perfect, and the ocean stretched out before us like a sheet of shimmering jewels. My wife and daughter were parked at the top of the hill, and we decided to call it a day.

We had clocked forty miles in seven hours and ten minutes.

A cold bath could wait. We immediately made our way to a local pizza parlor and fed our depleted bodies some much-needed calories. My legs were definitely beat up, but all in all I felt good about the two days we'd just completed. Knowing we "just" had a marathon to run on the final day was actually a relief. Imagine that.

Waking up on this third day was definitely tougher than the day before. My legs felt like someone had tied them in knots and dropped me from a three-story building. You've heard the saying, "Run over by a truck." Well, my entire body could relate. My mind was exhausted. The soreness and fatigue, however, I could handle. I was just happy that there was no apparent sign of an "overuse" injury.

The plan was for a later start the next morning. We would have time to stretch and calm our bodies down. We would have time for a good meal and plenty of prerun hydration.

The goal for the day was to run into San Luis Obispo from the backside of Arroyo Grande. We would then circle our way back into Pismo Beach. This was a scenic route highlighting the beautiful Edna Valley, and I was looking forward to it. Why not enjoy the bounties of Mother Nature while we were stretching our own physical and mental boundaries? This run measured approximately twenty-six miles, and it was an odd feeling that twenty-six miles didn't feel like too big of a day.

We took off at a leisurely pace, a pace slightly slower than the ones we set the previous two days. Once we warmed up, however, and had six miles under our belts, our legs began to feel better.

There was something about ultra-running that I was coming to realize. When you keep moving, your body gets into a rhythm and your legs actually feel good. It's like you reach new levels when you push through those uncomfortable times. The body has this natural reactive response. Stopping, on the other hand, shuts the body down. Muscles get tight and getting back in the groove is difficult. This was important information leading up to Limitless, and I planned to keep it in the back of mind.

Once we hit the fifteen-mile mark, I started to feel very strong. As limited and unfamiliar as my ultra-running experience was, I was a bit surprised that I felt this good at mile one hundred for the weekend. I started to put together a few surges. I would run hard for four or five minutes and then settle back into a comfortable pace for several minutes. I did this for about five miles and was pleasantly surprised at the result: the surges didn't tire me out, but actually added to my comfort level.

Hickey and I took a short break at the twenty-mile mark just outside of Avila Beach. My brother was filming this part of the run, and I told him, "I feel very good right now. I am actually a bit surprised."

"You're learning what the body can do," he replied. "Not many of us get to feel that."

We set out again, and a rather astounding revelation hit me twenty-one miles into the day's run, the one hundred and tenth mile of the weekend. "Dig deeper, Justin," I said aloud to myself. "You have more."

I continued to push. My body was tired and my legs were sore, but somehow I was able to dig deeper into an unexpected reservoir of strength. I learned something that day, a metaphor for life and living as a whole: "We must find the strength to keep pushing and dig deep in the toughest of times."

I absolutely killed the next five miles. I was actually running and running fast. My heart rate was low. I had a smooth rhythm. I was very controlled.

It came to me then: "If we are willing to dig deep inside of ourselves, we have the ability to push even harder. We have more strength, more drive, and more determination than we ever imagined. But the question is, are we willing to dig deep enough to find that inner strength?"

Digging that deep is hard because it's uncomfortable. But we all have the ability to overcome this discomfort. This inner strength alone will create a determined mindset that will drive us to our goals. I'm convinced of it.

"Do not be afraid to challenge yourself."

This is a message I share with all of my clients; it's also one of the strongest messages I can share with you. Do not be afraid to step outside of your comfort zone. Do not be afraid to push a little harder. You will truly see what you can do when you allow yourself to break down those limitations and push beyond your boundaries.

This brutal preparation for Limitless was all about breaking my own limits. I was finding myself. I was digging deep. Running these long, crazy distances was doing that for me. With every run, I was finding a new piece of whom I was as a human being. I was becoming physically, mentally, and spiritually stronger. I was exploring new emotions. I was finding an evolved way of life, and I was motivated to share this new way of life with others.

Our training camp came to an end at the iconic Splash Café in Pismo Beach. We finished the day at twenty-six miles almost to the number. After running 115 miles over a three-day span, we arrived to a crowd of people waiting in line for a bowl of the café's famous clam chowder. No one realized what we had just done. That wasn't important. We were ecstatic. New limits had been broken.

My body was sore, but my mind and heart were energized. We finished with a sense of confidence. We were ready to take on our Limitless goal of three hundred miles in one hundred hours. Hickey, Jim, Josh, and I found a table, sat, and took it all in. These were moments we would long cherish. We laughed. We shared our stories from the weekend. And we talked about the next step. The Limitless journey was arriving. We were ready for the ride.

That famous clam chowder tasted so good!

CHAPTER 10

....

DAYS AWAY

My wife is my best friend. Let's start there.

Now let me tell you how we met. It's a very funny story that sets the stage for a relationship that has only gotten better with time.

It was a Saturday night. My brother Josh, my good friend Ira (more on him later), and I were sitting around my house contemplating what we wanted to do that night. Did we want to go out and experience Visalia nightlife at its best or stay home and do whatever it is that three guys do when they're hanging out?

The latter didn't sound all that appealing, so we all agreed that we would grab "one" beer at the infamous Double LL Steakhouse. "And tonight," Josh said, "we'll let the girls come up to us."

Confident talk, I suppose, but we were all single at the time, and it wasn't like we were expecting to meet the loves of our lives that night.

We were three beers into the evening when a group of unfamiliar girls came walking into the bar. We Visalians recognize when new girls arrive in the bar. When it happens, it's worth taking note. But again, we were "waiting for them to come up to us."

I spotted Stephanie right away. She had long brown hair that framed a beautiful face and a challenging, mischievous smile. She was wearing cowgirl boots with sparkles and a country belt buckle that was meant to be noticed.

My brother Josh saw me looking. He said, "There you go, Justin," nodding his head in Stephanie's direction.

Next thing we knew, they were coming our way. Turns out they were celebrating a bachelorette party for one of their friends.

"We're on a scavenger hunt," one of them said.

"What's on your list?" Ira wanted to know.

"We need to ask a stranger for a piggyback ride."

Yup, I was that stranger for Stephanie. C'mon, meeting my soon-to-be wife at Double LL? Does that really happen? Well, it happened for me. Want proof? We have a photograph of me giving Stephanie a piggyback ride hanging in the family room of our house. It's one of my prized possessions.

We started dating. A year later, we were engaged. A year after that, we tied the knot. We have been married six years now, and every day is better than the last.

From the get-go, Stephanie knew I was "kind of" a fitness fanatic. Ok, "kind of" is a bit of an understatement. She knew she was dating a guy that had a deep passion for fitness, health, and positive living. I had only done one triathlon when we met. During our first year together, I began training for my first Olympic-distance event. The whole "endurance lifestyle" was still new to us both. Before children, it was easy to plan a weekend around an event. It was two lovebirds traveling to a triathlon, hanging out, having fun, and enjoying each other's company.

Stephanie was and is still my number-one fan. At every event I can hear her calling, "C'mon babe." It means the world to me knowing she is supporting me. To date, she has seen me complete over sixty events. When I first came to her with the idea of running three hundred miles in one hundred hours, I put it this way: "I am embarking on something big. And I want your blessing. If

I'm going to do this, I need to know that you're on board 100 percent. Otherwise, it's not worth doing."

From day one, she was all in. Well, maybe deep down she was apprehensive, but she didn't show any signs of backing down. I knew I needed her by my side every "step" of the way.

Some people see Stephanie as a quiet, slightly subdued woman. Don't let that fool you. She is totally present. She is very intelligent. She is hard working. She speaks her mind. She is also one of the most beautiful, loving, and compassionate people I know. Our personalities may be different, but we connect on so many levels. As important as anything, we respect each other. She allows me to be me, and I her. Our relationship has surely had its ups and downs, but we have always managed to work out our issues. The result, I believe, is a stronger, more supportive couple.

Our first child was born on February 15, 2011. We named her Olivia JoJo. I call her JoJo. From day one, JoJo was our princess. She lights up our lives in every way possible. Having a child changes things in the most spectacular way. Yes, there are more responsibilities. Yes, your focus changes. Yes, your cost of living goes through the roof. Yet the joy I get from this little person is without peer. I look forward to seeing JoJo every day; I look forward to watching her grow and change and being a part of every moment.

A year and half after JoJo was born, Stephanie and I found ourselves expecting again. As I described early, we tragically lost Inspire at thirty-five weeks. But with tragedy comes triumph. Five months later, we were pregnant again. On February 11, 2014, we gave birth to a beautiful baby girl named Bobbi Jo. These two girls are the sparks that make every day magical. Stephanie and I cherish every second we have with them.

Olivia JoJo had just turned two as our preparations for the Limitless run were gaining momentum, and she knew that Daddy was up to something big.

Before we knew it, we were a week from departure and still had so much to do. Stephanie was five months pregnant and had a two-year-old to tend to: job one. Job two was driving one of the RVs that would follow me every step of the way. Stephanie was also in charge of food prep. This was an integral component in the success of our expedition. Since I would be burning between nine thousand and thirteen thousand calories a day, food consumption was a priority. The grocery store trip the night before we packed the RV was an event all its own. Lunchmeat, Cliff bars, fruit, Eggo waffles, eggs, milk, bread, peanut butter, chocolate chip cookies, Gatorade, canned soups, coffee, trail mix, and who knows what else. Food for four days and eight people.

The week leading up to the Limitless launch was also filled with interviews with the local newspaper and several radio stations, the taping of a morning television show, and a constant barrage of social media. I also had my normal business responsibilities to tend to. We packed our clothes. We readied our food. We tuned our vehicles. Josh and his team prepared their camera equipment.

I made a conscious effort to pack as many hours of sleep as I could into the days leading up to the run because we all knew that sleep would be a limited commodity over the next four-and-a-half days. On the other hand, I only ran a few times in the week leading up to the event. I wanted to keep my legs limber and moving, but I also wanted to be 100 percent going into the run.

"Tapering" for an event of this nature is different than it is for a triathlon or a shorter race. For a triathlon, I would generally maintain the frequency of my training but reduce the training volume. I would also increase the intensity. So, for example, instead of a normal 3,500-yard workout in the pool, a "taper" workout would be more like 1,600 yards with some fast 50s to stay sharp.

Overall, training volume during the week leading up to an "A" race is reduced by approximately fifty percent. This allows full recovery from all the training stress applied in the weeks and months before the actual event. In any case, the goal was to keep my body sharp without overstressing it.

Tapering for a three-hundred-mile run was something new to me. I had no point of reference.

Two weeks before my departure, my initial plan was to reduce my weekly running volume by fifty percent. The week before, my plan was to run two or three times for no more than forty-five minutes. I call it "casual running." The goal is to be as strong and fit as possible going into the run.

I was surprisingly calm the week before the run. We were all so busy and pre-occupied that I think my mind forgot to get nervous. Deep down, of course, I could not help but wonder what the run would be like. And, as you will see, the experience went much deeper than expected and on levels I could never have anticipated.

My brother Josh and I had a routine. He would say things like, "Dude, you're about to run three hundred miles. Are you ready for this?"

My very methodical, unemotional answer would always be the same: "Yeah man, I got this."

The Monday before we departed was a very long day. A television crew arrived at CFA at 4:30 that morning for an interview. It took all morning. Midday I was able to hurry home to rest my eyes, but the afternoon was nonstop business. Monday night we packed the RV and shared some family time.

That night, my dad asked me the very same thing Josh had been asking me for weeks: "Are you ready for this?"

I don't know why I fielded his question any differently than I might have Josh's, but my nerves got to me for the first time when it came from my dad. The anxiety was real. Very real.

CHAPTER 11

AN OVERWHELMING MORNING

Tuesday morning arrived. And while the anxiety still remained to a degree, excitement and readiness were the dominant emotions once my feet hit the floor.

I was physically and mentally prepared. I had gotten a surprisingly good night's sleep and woke up around 4:15 a.m., a little later than my normal wake-up time. I was rested and ready for the big day and an even bigger week ahead. But this, I recognized, was an expedition. I planned to take it day by day, moment by moment.

I enjoyed my shower, knowing it would be my last for a while; yes, the RV had a shower, but no, it would not be nearly as relaxing as this one.

The crew—or most of them—met at the house at 5:15 am. The vibes were positive, the conversation casual. We ate breakfast. I had two scrambled eggs (140 calories) and a banana (seventy-five calories); light, but filling enough. I had learned that my stomach reacted differently during ultra-running than it did during a half marathon or shorter races. Keep it light. Allow the stomach to digest the food quickly. Eat more often.

After breakfast, I used the foam roller and some light movements to loosen up. This was my normal pre-workout routine. Ten minutes of foam rolling and a five-minute dynamic warm-up to prepare the body for the work ahead.

Rocky Ciseneros, our team's physical therapist, showed up around 5:30 a.m., and we chatted as I was warming up. Rocky has a doctorate in physical therapy and works at a local facility. His main clientele are runners. I grew up with Rocky. We went to the same high school, played on the same football and soccer teams, and now he is an active member of the Visalia Triathlon Club. Rocky is the expert in our area when it comes to sports injuries. I completely trust his expertise.

We had fully packed the RV the night before, so all was left was to pack up Olivia JoJo and her most cherished toys. She would be with us the entire week. I wanted this; I needed this. I knew it would be tough for Stephanie—she had already taken on a ton of responsibilities for this crazy journey of mine—but I knew JoJo would put a smile on my face every time I saw her. She would be my secret, uplifting weapon.

As I shut the door behind us, I probably didn't realize the magnitude of what was about to happen over the next four-and-a-half days, but I did have a moment where I thought it very likely that I would come back a changed person.

We stopped for gas, ice, and a few last food items at Four Seasons Handy Mart, a neighborhood place owned by our good friends Jim and Mike Means. I later found out that Jim paid for everything that morning, his gift to our Limitless adventure. I couldn't believe it. It was humbling to say the least.

As we headed for downtown Visalia, I was amped up. We had spent the past few weeks promoting the start of the run and had been asking people to join us for a one-mile jog around downtown Visalia. We had posted announcements in the newspaper, with Facebook posts and emails, and via word of mouth. We had no idea how many people would actually show up. Yes, we have a wonderful running community in town, and yes, the people are as genuine as they are positive, but I had no idea if anyone would actually show up.

I had invited all of the local running clubs; the Visalia Runners Club was the most established of these groups, having been around since the 80s, but there were an abundance of other smaller groups that I hoped would respond. I knew that The Mavericks, a local group of runners, were definitely excited for my run, and they had shown tremendous support and encouragement over the past few weeks, so I was confident they would be there. I had my fingers crossed.

It was still dark when we arrived, but there was already a crowd of people milling around the starting line. I couldn't believe it. It was an overwhelming feeling. A cheer went up as we pulled into the parking lot. I had tears in my eyes as I jumped down and saw all the smiling faces. I tried my best to say hello to everyone individually and to express my gratitude. Nothing could have been more heartfelt.

Probably my most memorable conversation that morning was with my good friend Brian Hyde. At 6'7", Brian soared over most of the crowd and, standing next to yours truly who is a good foot shorter, we probably looked a bit like the "odd couple." But Brian was completely sincere when he said, "This is truly inspirational, Justin. I am not sure you recognize how much the Limitless project has inspired people."

He was right. At that very moment, I wasn't fully aware of the deep motivation the project was providing. Of course, I had hoped as much, but it wasn't until later, when other people approached me with their stories, that I realized our message was indeed getting out and doing its job.

It was emotional to see the support that first morning. People cared, and it showed.

I spent a few minutes addressing the crowd. It gave me a chance to express my gratitude to everyone for their support and to bow our heads in prayer. It was emotional and uplifting.

At 6:30, we gathered thirty or so runners together and the countdown started. Everyone in attendance was shouting, "Five, four, three, two, one." Horns sounded and we were off. This was one of the coolest sights of the entire trip. There we were, runners of all shapes, sizes, and skill levels running through downtown Visalia, spreading optimism, inspiration, community, and wellness.

The goal of the Limitless project was to spread the message to people regardless of their fitness level that "anything is possible," and that truly believing in yourself is the key to optimal living. The start of the run was the perfect compliment to this goal. It was much more than I could have dreamt for. Positive energy, wide smiles, infectious laughter, a true sense of community. At that exact moment, with Stephanie and JoJo looking on, life was perfect.

The sun was inching its way along the horizon, a shock of orange and gold painting the sky, as we made our way down the road for our "victory lap." It was a beautiful sight.

When our loop was completed, a cheer went up and Team Limitless was officially launched. Five runners, one bicyclist, an RV piloted by my wife, and a camera crew directed by my brother made our way out of Visalia.

I knew one thing: I couldn't run three hundred miles in one hundred hours alone. My pace runners were an indispensable component to this adventure. At the outset, I had five of the very best, as much for their friendship and inspiration as for their running: Sean Taylor, James Wilson, Salina Marroquin, Steve Juarez, and Eric Galvan. All were "runners" except Eric. We'd met sixteen weeks earlier. Eric worked as a newspaper reporter for the local paper. He became intrigued with the Limitless project and wrote a series of articles that really helped spread the word and inspired participation in both the run and the foundation we were supporting.

Eric had long lived a sedentary lifestyle. He saw what we were doing and wanted a change. He started blogging; the blog talked about his new lifestyle goals and how his involvement with Limitless was providing motivation. He set a goal to run with us on the first portion of the race, and to that end, he busted his butt training. When all was said and done, the proof, as they say, was in the pudding: here he was running side by side with the five of us as the first leg of our journey opened up in front of us, and it never occurred to us that he wouldn't be able to hold up his end.

And then there was Sean Taylor. His was an equally inspirational story that he describes here in his own words:

I was a very active eight year old. Almost every day of the year you could find me running or rollerblading, skateboarding or playing baseball. One day, almost without warning, I began to experience a lot of pain near my left hip and behind my knee. It took doctors four months to finally diagnose me with Legg-Perthes, a childhood condition that affects the hip where the thighbone (femur) and pelvis meet in a ball-and-socket joint. At first, the doctors thought I had sprained my hip. But it was much more serious than that. My hip had actually "died" due to poor blood circulation. I was told that walking would be a chore, and that running and other sports were out of the picture.

Life changed for my family and me that day. I was placed in an A-frame brace and spent my entire third grade wearing it. Eight months! When that did not work, I had complete reconstructive hip surgery, building a shelf out of part of my pelvis in hopes that a new hip head would grow back. I spent three months in a thirty-nine-pound body cast. I had to have physical therapy for one year and had to relearn how to walk at the age of ten. I never told anyone how much pain I was in. Suffice to say it was way over a "10." Sometimes just getting out of bed took real courage, but I never gave up. When I was in seventh grade, I ran my first cross-country race. I ran cross-country and track in high school for four years and was featured in Runner's World magazine my senior year as their superstar athlete of the month. I have since run three marathons, multiple half marathons, and have for many years represented the Tulare County Sheriff's Department by running a leg in the Baker-to-Vegas team relay. I recently completed a four-day bike tour with my brother Kile down the central California coast.

As I trained for Team Limitless, I reflected on some of the limits I'd overcome since my childhood and realized that the only person who could impose limits on me was me.

Even before the Limitless run commenced that early morning, I realized that it was inspiring people to break free of their own limits. People were out there achieving massive goals, and Limitless was a platform to highlight their endeavors.

I realized something else that morning. This was not just about me running three hundred miles in one hundred hours. It was about this awesome community coming together, sharing their passions, testing their boundaries, living healthy, and finding themselves.

When all was said and done, this was a team event.

CHAPTER 12

....

LET'S RUN

Day 1: Visalia to Oildale

Making our way through our hometown was clearly one of the highlights of the Limitless experience, but now that the hoopla was behind us, it was time to run.

We had a motorcycle cop escort us to the city limits. We ran down Caldwell Avenue, a popular stretch of road that pipelines Visalia to Farmersville and right into Exeter. Local cyclists use Caldwell Avenue as they make their way into the hills of Yokohl Valley and beyond. This is where the police officer bade us farewell, and we were officially on our way out of town. The first twelve miles went seemingly in the blink of an eye as we made our way through Farmersville and Exeter. The energy driving the entire team was positive, the conversation was stimulating, and our pace over this first stretch was right around ten-minute miles. Comfortable, yet not overly aggressive.

We made a quick pit stop at a convenience store in Exeter to use the restroom and reapply sun block. It was only 8:30 and already we could predict warmer weather.

Going into the run, the weather had been almost fall-like: cool mornings and mid-70s in the afternoon. I had been checking weather forecasts regularly leading up to our launch, and sure enough, we were destined to be running during the five hottest days the area had seen so far since summer, upper 90s at times.

One TV reporter had even joked with me during one of our pre-race interviews, saying, "Do you know you will be running during the four hottest days of the month?"

I jokingly answered, "Makes for a great movie, right?"

After our pit stop, we got back into our rhythm again and found the adrenaline of our sendoff still pushing us forward. Our pace runners began to peel off at the twenty-mile marker. It was bittersweet saying our goodbyes, but it was also amazingly gratifying knowing these wonderful people had seen fit to be an integral part of Limitless. By the time we passed the thirty-mile mark, it was just Josh Hickey, Jim Barnes on his road bike, and me. Less my brother's camera crew and an occasional sighting of our RV, this would be our main crew over the next few days. If Josh and I expected a stretch of tranquility, it was short lived, because we had a bona fide storyteller in our midst. Jim Barnes had a story for every occasion. He completed over a hundred endurance events, and he had a story about every one of them. Sometimes two or three stories. And yes, we were destined to hear them all, and more often than not we were grateful for the distraction. It kept our minds moving and our spirits high, especially when we got deeper into the run and our bodies were beaten down. One of Jim's stories always served as the perfect salve and would inevitably stray us away from thinking about our physical despair.

You want Jim on your side. He is a happy-go-lucky guy whose positive vibe is contagious. His strong faith and spiritual guidance were something this journey needed. Jim was more than just the guy on the bike carrying our food. He was a spiritual blanket that kept us safe and out of harm's way.

As the country roads of Porterville opened up before us, the temperature escalated. We knew the worst of the heat was yet to come, so we did our best to focus on the moment at hand. Because Josh is bigger than me—actually quite a bit bigger than me—the heat hit him harder and his pace slowed slightly. He also sweats more than I do and therefore required more hydration. Because I was feeling good and running strong, I paced myself accordingly. This was the plan: I would set whatever pace I was comfortable with, and the others would do the same. I knew my pace runners were there for me and doing all they could to steady the ship. This wasn't a race. If a runner dropped too far behind and we needed to make an executive decision about whether he or she should continue on, we did what was best for everyone without tampering too significantly with the system we had laid out.

We were eight miles from our lunch break and on the outskirts of Porterville when we made a quick stop to fill our water bottles, wet our faces, and reapply sunscreen. I was in a good mood, joking around and laughing, and signaled to our support crew that "everything was all right" both physically and mentally. They would learn later that the minute my mood shifted and I became agitated, fatigue was setting in big time and it was time to regroup. Thirty-two miles into the run, however, I felt pretty darn strong.

Running into Porterville felt particularly good because it was our first official destination. It turned out to be a long spurt, however. The community college where we planned to stop for lunch was another five miles away, and those five miles proved to be long and arduous. The temperature continued to climb, and we were hitting the forty-mile mark for the day. My body was starting to fatigue.

I stripped off my shirt. I improvised a bandana and tied it around my head. My stomach began to cramp. Not the best situation for running, but we were almost to the Porterville campus. Later, Rocky, our consulting nutritionist, would determine that I was consuming too much synthetic sugar from gels, electrolyte drink mixes, and shot blocks. The answer was to cut way back on these products and to consume primarily solid foods moving forward and to drink plain old water for hydration. We also concluded that the intensity of the running was a contributing factor. Since my pace was slow—or at least slower than a triathlon or a half-marathon—my body was failing to utilize the quick sugars right away, and they would go straight to my gut. In contrast, the gels and synthetic sugars were not a problem when running a half marathon or triathlon, where the pace is higher and the sugars kick in immediately.

Josh had slipped behind me over the last few miles, and Jim was riding along with him just to make sure he was okay, so I ran alone over the last five miles.

When I hit the parking lot, there were a dozen people from Team in Training (an organization that raises money for the Leukemia and Lymphoma Foundation) cheering me on. I cannot tell you much I appreciated those cheers. My spirits had taken a hit over the last stretch of miles, so having the Team in Training supporters out there definitely gave me a much-needed boost.

My feet were already sore, so I quickly slipped off my shoes and plunged my feet in a bucket of ice-cold water. The relief was instantaneous.

Josh and Jim arrived about five minutes after I did, and it was a welcome sight. Stephanie made us grilled ham-and-cheese sandwiches, and it was one of the best meals I've ever eaten.

Breaks like this one would turn out to be lifesavers over the next four days. And though we tried our best not to overstay our welcome, a few minutes off our feet did wonders for our recovery and gave us the impetus to move forward again.

Before we did so, Rocky ran me through the numbers. He took my weight, measured my blood pressure, checked my heart rate, assessed my feet, and asked me four questions: "Are you pee-ing?" "What color is your pee?" "How is your mood?" "Anything I should know about?"

My answers apparently satisfied him, because he gave me a thumb's up to keep going.

The other positive news was that my good friend Eric Blain was also waiting for us when we arrived at the college. The plan was for Eric to run the next portion with us. I was looking forward to this. Eric is a great friend and training partner. He has a way of creating conversations while we run that invariably make the time go by just a little bit faster.

Our ten minutes were almost over when I remembered to call Kent Moore, my public relations manager. The plan was to touch base throughout the day with updates on our progress, and then he would post the news on my Facebook page. I cannot tell you how encouraging it was to read the comments and messages from my Facebook friends supporting this journey. The messages were both awesome and humbling. Every one of them provided motiva-tion. Every one of them kept me going.

"Be aware of the chair."

This was one of Josh Hickey's invaluable pieces of ultra-run-ning advice. Simply put, once you decide to sit down during an ultra-distance run, it is hard as hell to get back up. "Your body will inevitably rebel against you if you're not prepared."

I didn't know it at the time, but as the run progressed, Josh's warning would ring ever truer and it would get harder and harder to "pull my body out of the chair."

Our Porterville stop wasn't so bad, however. My body was tight and my feet were certainly sore, but I managed to pop out of that chair and call the troops to arms. Time to run.

We left the Porterville College campus and were immediately in the country. If I thought it was hot earlier, now we were running with temperatures broaching the upper 90s. And since we were on black pavement, it made for even hotter conditions. You could feel the heat penetrating the pavement. The sun was beaming. Sweat poured off us like buckets of rainwater. Hydration was, to say the least, critical. We had to pay attention to even the smallest sign of dehydration: if you stopped sweating, if it had been a while since your last pee break, or if you felt even the slightest bit lightheaded.

Staying on top of this component was vital. Once dehydration sets in, heat exhaustion—and even worse, heat stroke—can follow. Rocky was relentless; he couldn't say it often enough: "Drink more water." It was like a never-ending mantra: drink more water.

Immediately into this next portion, we noticed Hickey dropping back from what was really a conservative 10.5-minute mile pace. At Jim's encouragement and Rocky's insistence, he decided to hang out in the RV for a few hours. It was a smart decision. There was no reason to test fate. I knew Josh wanted to run the entire three hundred miles with me—we both hoped for that— but we also knew that there might be times where circumstances forced us to split up. Hickey is a very smart runner and more experienced than me; I would need his expertise the entire run, so resting and allowing his body and mind to recover were crucial to our success.

I knew he was disappointed. I was disappointed not having him by my side. But the break was necessary. One, it was prudent for right now. And two, it was necessary so that he could continue with us later.

So now it was Eric and me running, with Jim cycling next to us. We made our way to Ducor, a very small city just thirteen miles south of Porterville. It was here that we merged onto Highway 65. We would stay on 65 for the remainder of the afternoon and into the evening.

I wasn't thinking about how many miles we had run or how long we would stay on Highway 65. I didn't want to think one hundred miles down the road. I didn't want to think even fifty miles down the road. I set small goals for myself: looking no more than ten or fifteen miles up the road. Getting to Ducor was a goal met, but I also dropped into a serious low spot right about the same time. My mood ebbed. I became subdued and quiet. Conversation ceased and we ran in silence.

In ultra-running, you can tell when you've entered a battle zone. Silence takes over. Talking ceases. Little things start to annoy. The mind goes virtually blank. The legs keep churning. In time, hopefully, the low spot passes.

One thing is certain, when I hit a wall or drop into a low spot, I make sure to communicate to my crew how I'm feeling. That puts them on the alert. They watch. They observe. They decide if they need to take action.

In this case, I pulled my hat very low on my head, my eyes seeing only a few steps in front of me, my mind focused on the here and now.

"One step at a time." This was my mantra when low spots hit. "One step at a time."

This particular low spot only lasted a few miles, but it was a small taste of what would come later in the journey.

We stopped for a quick break right before we turned onto Highway 65. All I wanted was a good dousing of cold water over my head. I washed my face in cold water as well, and this woke me up. A few laughs livened up the mood, and my energy sparked.

Rocky blasted me with a quick round of questions. The answers revealed that my last bathroom break was two hours ago, so he stressed fluid intake at this stop. By this time, hunger was definitely starting to get to me. With the extreme calorie loss that running all day brings, it was difficult to manage the times when I just got plain hungry. In a moment of inspiration, my mom bought a batch of tacos from a taco truck, but I could only manage one. I was hungry, but for some reason nothing sounded too inviting.

Eric and I continued running. When we hit Highway 65 and turned south toward Bakersfield, we were greeted by heavy traffic, aggressive drivers, and a very narrow shoulder. It was dangerous, but we had to move forward. As the miles ticked away, the sun slipped closer and closer toward the horizon, and a tinge of orange and gold washed across the sky. The country fields to the east swayed in a gentle breeze. It was a pretty cool scene, and I took a moment to enjoy it. My brother Josh's camera caught the whole thing on tape.

I glanced at my watch. It was 6:30. With the setting sun came the most ideal running conditions we had experienced all day, and Eric and I savored the moment. We took a short break to put our headlamps and reflectors on and pressed ahead.

Initially, our goal was Bakersfield or bust. But as I started calculating the miles, I decided to run until 10:30 p.m. At our current speed, that would leave us thirteen miles shy of Bakersfield. Not ideal, but satisfactory.

Running Highway 65 at night probably was not the smartest thing to do. The four-foot shoulder was sketchy at best as cars, pickups, and big rigs barreled down the road as if their last meal awaited them. Worse, our headlamps seemed to draw the attention of the drivers headed our way and cause them to veer even closer to the shoulder. There were definitely some close calls along the way, made more scary yet by the fact that deep fatigue was causing Eric and me to get a bit blurry-headed.

Except for Jim on his trusty bike, our companion vehicles had to move down the road. The last couple hours passed in a fog. It's hard to explain, but running for fifteen hours in one day creates a delusional feeling. I was very aware of my surroundings, yet my mind had essentially shut down.

It was like running in a trance; that's how tired I was. We took short breaks every forty-five minutes to sip soda that provided miniscule bursts of energy that pushed us a few more miles at a time. By the time 10:00 p.m. rolled around, it took some real guts to say, "Let's go for thirty more minutes," but those were exactly the words I heard coming from my mouth. Thankfully, Eric didn't complain.

We mixed short periods of walking with a slow run, and a few more miles ticked away. I was sleepy and ready to call it a night. My goal was to hit as close to eighty miles on this first day as possible, but we only clocked sixty-seven. That would have to do. At that point, the best decision was to grab some sleep and get back after it in the morning.

We found some space right off Highway 65 just outside of Oildale, a small city outside Bakersfield. There was just enough room for our two RVs and the three other vehicles tracking our progress.

What a day it had been. Sixteen hours of straight running! Sixty-seven miles was by far the farthest I had ever run. It was unforgettable from start to finish. The crowds who bade us good luck in the morning. My wife, daughter, and mother staying close by in their RV. Josh and his crew making a movie of the entire thing. My pace runners keeping me on point. Jim, Rocky, and so many wonderful men and women lending their expertise and support.

To our complete and total satisfaction, there were four hot pizzas awaiting our arrival, and we completely devoured them. Never has something as simple as a takeout pizza tasted so good.

We were also happy to see my good friend Tyler Baxley when we arrived. Tyler planned to run with us the next morning. He was stoked about the Limitless adventure, and we were excited to see yet another fresh runner to pull us closer to our goal.

While we ate and soaked our tired feet, we gave Tyler a run-down on the day and gave him some idea of what to expect the next morning.

Once I sat down in a chair, my body stiffened up quickly. My feet were already swollen, so I immediately stuck them in ice to help with the deep inflammation and swelling. After icing, I lay on the table so Rocky could do some light manual therapy. As soon as this stretching session was completed, I went in the RV and took a shower; I never knew a shower, no matter how small or lacking in pressure, could feel so good.

I was cooked after that. Bedtime.

I should have slept like a log given what I had put my body through that day, but I didn't. I tossed and turned all night. Not only was my body aching all over, but we had parked so close to the highway that the big rigs rumbling past shook our RV like a rag doll in the hands of a two year old. Before I knew it, 5:00 a.m. had arrived and it was time to go again.

Day 1: 67 miles

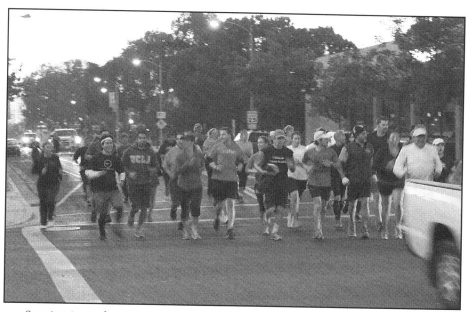

Starting in my hometown of Visalia, CA, we started with a mile 1 "victory lap" around downtown with a positive group of supporters.

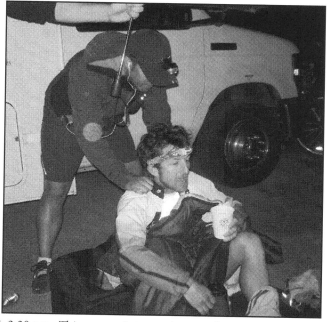

Mile 265, 3:30 am. This was an intense pit stop where I was beyond physically and mentally tired.

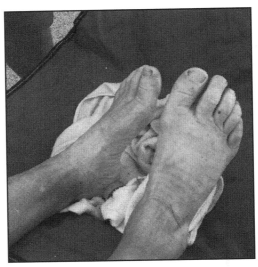

My feet at mile 170.

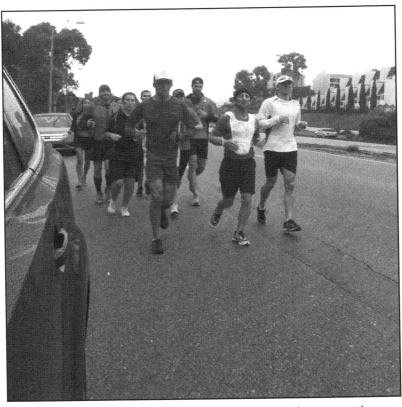

Running down Highway 1 in Malibu. Thirteen miles to go with a great group of runners.

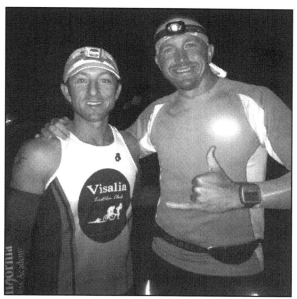

Morning of Day 2 with my #1 pace runner, Josh Hickey. We were in good spirits.

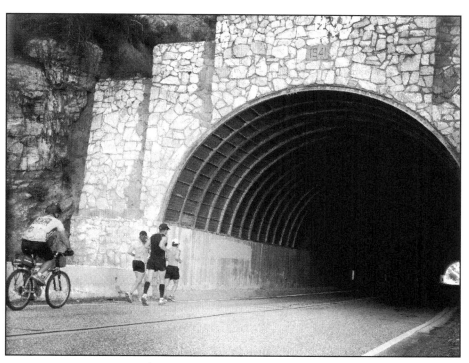

Mile 200, running the Angeles Forest.

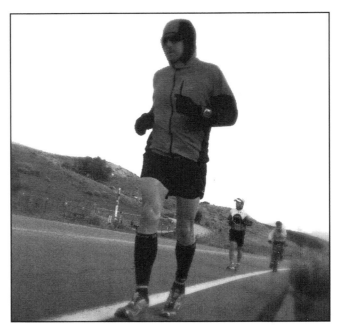

Morning of Day 4, climbing into the Angeles Forest.
It was a cold and windy morning.

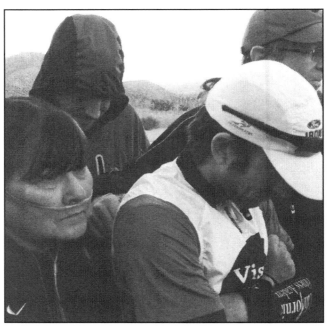

Morning of Day 4, before we started. Knowing we still had 110 miles to run,
I was subdued and depressed.

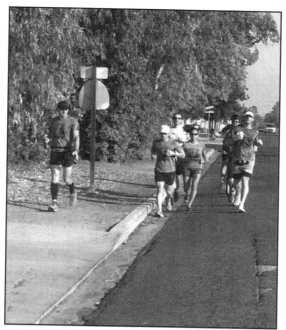

Day 1, mile 15, running with my pace runners.

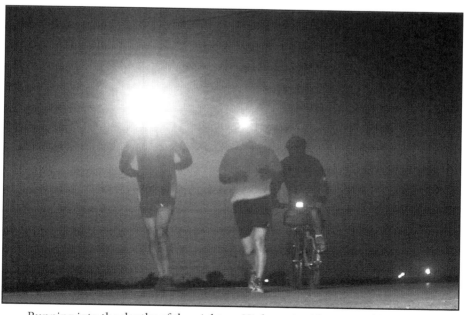

Running into the depths of the night on Highway 1 with my good friend Ira, and of course Jim on his trusty bike.

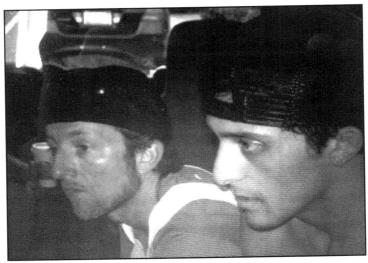

Mile 290, my deepest hole of the run. Ira and I staring in a trance.
We were both at our physical and mental limits.

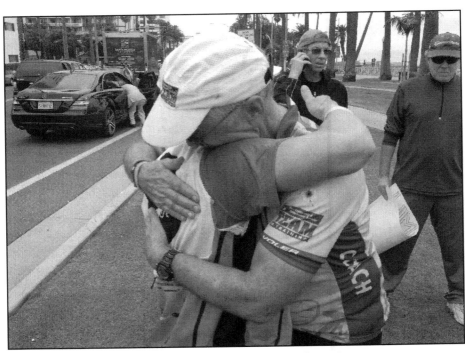

An emotional embrace at the finish with Jim Barnes.
He was by my side for 300 miles on a bike.

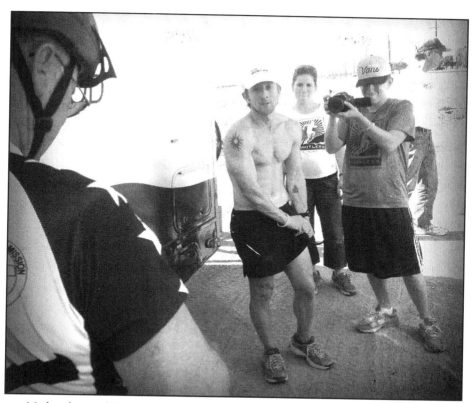

My brother Josh had a camera in my face the entire run. I didn't mind though.

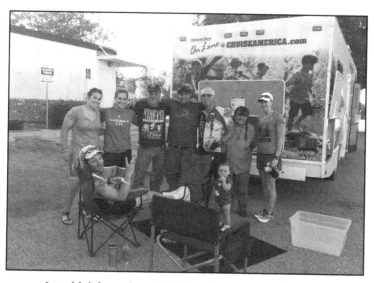

I couldn't have done it without these group of people.

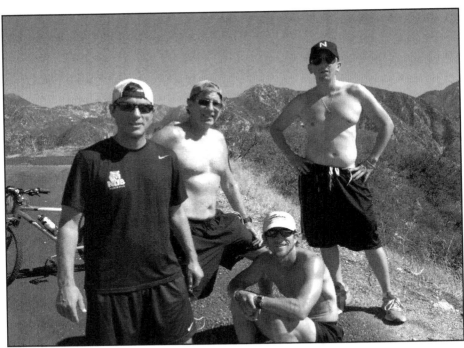

An epic experience, peaking the summit of the Angeles Forest with my two brothers and my dad. I will never forget this moment.

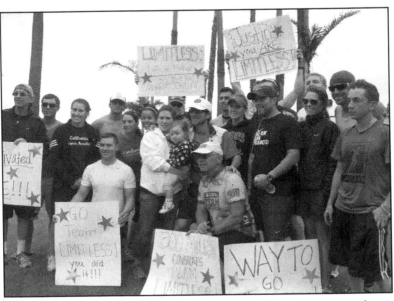

The finish! Mile 300! This was a moment I did not want to end.

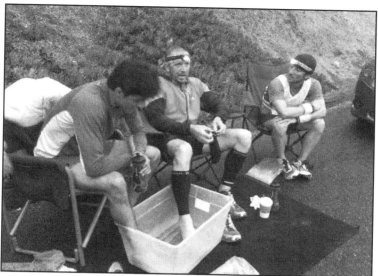

After a long night of running, we were in high spirits at mile 280, sitting along Highway 1. Ira and Hickey icing their feet, I'm just chilling', we laughed!

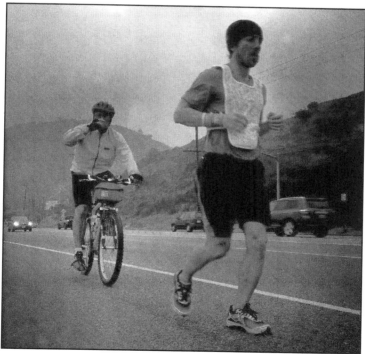

Mile 295, Jim by my side as I put one foot in front of the other. I was almost there!

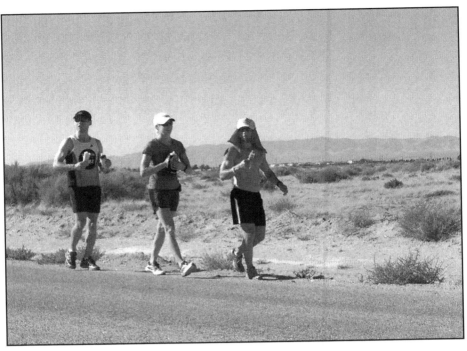

Mojave Desert run with Landon and Lindsey.

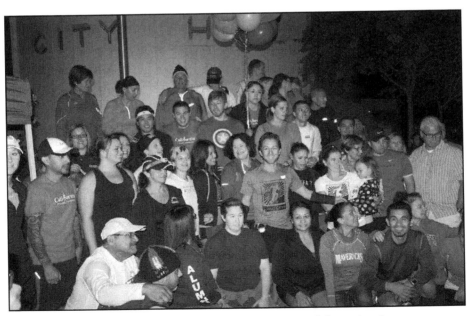

It was an overwhelming morning before we started this epic adventure.
I was humbled and very appreciative of the support.

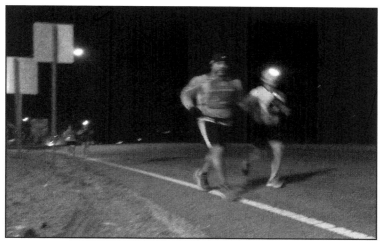

Day 3 night. We had been running for 13 hours and we still had about 3 to go!
I was tired and hungry.

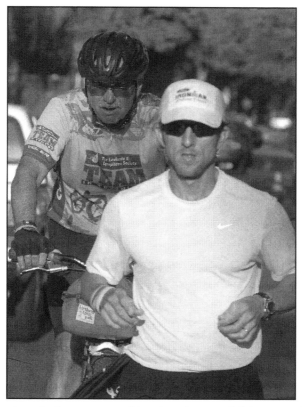

Running into the busy streets of Los Angeles. We didn't expect the chaos
but we adjusted and continued our journey.

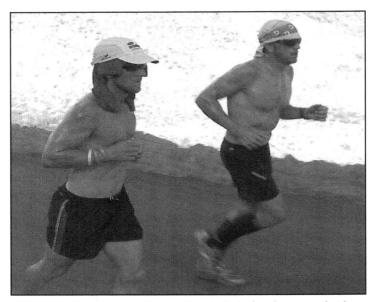

Hickey and I battling the heat and the hills before hitting Tehachapi.

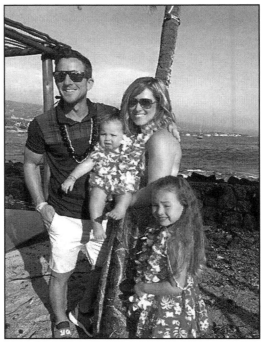

My Family

CHAPTER 13

....

ON THE ROAD AGAIN

Day 2: Oildale to Tehachapi

I am a morning person. Most mornings I am up before 4:30 a.m. Mondays, Wednesdays, and Fridays, my alarm goes off at 3:55, and I am at my gym an hour later preparing for the day ahead. Our first clients arrive at 5:00. I like to be wide awake, fully energized, and ready to go the minute they walk through the door.

Each individual workout is already written on the board, and I spend upwards of ten minutes on mobility and flexibility work getting prepared.

Our clients pay for the best possible service, and if my staff and I aren't giving them energy and motivation, no matter the time spent, then I am not doing my job.

Waking up early has been something I have done since my paperboy days. This is not to say that I don't enjoy and cherish those morning when I get to "sleep in." Let me put it a different way: I enjoy and cherish the days when an alarm doesn't wake me up. On these days, I am still up by 6:30 or 6:45, and that's sleeping in for me.

This first night in the RV was different. With my wife, daughter, and teammates close by, the ringing of my phone alarm began infiltrating my dreams. I was obviously in a very deep sleep, because it took a good two minutes for me to realize that the alarm was the real deal and I needed to wake up. It took me a lot less time than that to realize how sore and stiff my body was. An inconsistent and far-from-satisfying sleep did not help matters.

It was 5:15. Our Day 2 goal was to get going around 5:45 a.m. Within minutes, everyone on our crew was up and moving around. I heard someone making coffee. Thank goodness.

I assessed the damage from yesterday. Besides the usual stiffness, I was pretty good, physically speaking. The swelling in my feet was probably my biggest concern, but all and all I felt encouraged.

We ate breakfast—two Eggo waffles with jam and a banana—and started to ponder the day ahead. We were ten miles from Bakersfield, so getting there became our initial goal. We wanted to get an early start to finish our run on Highway 65 with minimal traffic.

I drank some fluids to start my hydration for the day and finished putting on my gear. Since we were setting out before sunrise, Tyler, Josh, and I began our trek with headlamps and reflectors. The good news was that the traffic was light, which made for peaceful running.

As the sun started to rise, the scene to our left was nothing short of spectacular. The sunlight hit the bronzed-colored foothills of Bakersfield, and they burst with glittering color and subtle texture. It was a sight to behold.

We knew were in the middle of "Oildale" because we were surrounded with oil rigs yo-yoing up and down. It was a picture-perfect depiction of the industrial Central Valley country. The three of us were chugging at a nice clip, and the first ten miles flew by. Good conversation, some laughs, and the perfect temperature. Before we knew it, we merged onto James Way, a relatively peaceful concourse leading into Bakersfield. No more Highway

65! Hallelujah! It was a relief to be off such a busy thoroughfare, especially one that seemed to go on forever.

We paused at mile eighteen—mile eighty-six for the entire trip—and took a short break. We ate, applied sunscreen, and rested our legs.

The night before, I had been in contact with a Bakersfield television crew that wanted to do a story on the project. I was excited. The publicity would be a boon for the Limitless project and our charities. We were supposed to meet with their crew on the outskirts of the city, but it hadn't worked out. So after our break, we made plans to meet at a local church four miles farther on and do a quick interview.

We arrived at the church parking lot an hour later, and the television camera crew and interviewer were waiting. I answered a few questions and talked about the project. The camera crew filmed some footage. They planned to run the story on the evening news, and I was thrilled for the exposure.

Twenty minutes later, we were waving goodbye to our team and back at it.

The weather began heating up, and our running intervals got progressively shorter; this was to be expected. We needed more frequent breaks to stay cool and ice our legs and feet. We decided to take short breaks every three or four miles just to rinse our faces, hydrate, and eat. It was a good pace, especially running through East Bakersfield, where industrial buildings, dogs barking, and destitute land painted the landscape. Unique and a little disquieting.

Despite the setting, we took another break to rest and hydrate; my body was also telling me that I needed food. We set up our "off-the-road aid station," including RVs, escort cars, and camera crew, sat down, and chilled for a bit. The heat was already making its presence felt, and the concrete jungle of East Bakersfield didn't help.

We knew we had plenty of running to do that day, so staying fueled, hydrated, and cool were crucial. There we were, just beyond a light industrial park, sprawled along the sidewalk, with wet towels on our heads, food in our hands, and legs propped up. It was an amusing sight, and the curious looks we received from passing motorists said it all.

I was tired and needed to rest my eyes for a few minutes, but overall my spirits were high, and we were enjoying each other's company.

After a fifteen-minute break, it was time to push on. Maybe we had paused a bit too long, because I found it a bit tougher to get up and get moving this time. Stiff did not adequately describe it. The solution? We started with some walking to get the legs moving, then the walk turned into a slow jog, which eventually morphed into our normal running pace.

We finally made our way to the Edison Highway, a country thoroughfare that runs parallel to Highway 58. While Highway 58 is a popular access route between Bakersfield and Las Vegas, it is not nearly as conducive to running as was the raggedy, winding Edison Highway, and we were all glad to be on it.

Tyler and Josh were prime running partners. Free spirited, motivated, and selfless; you couldn't ask for better characteristics in your running mates. With Jim on his bike for moral support, it was hard to do better.

As well as the three of us had been doing all day, we hit the wall at mile twenty-five for the day. My body and mind started to go flat. The heat sapped my energy and took a huge bite out of the stamina that I relied on in such a big way.

Hitting the wall is not fun. Every runner who has ever gone through it will attest to that. The negative emotions started bombarding you from every direction, and the mind starts to play tricks on you.

You manage these low spots with cold towels, calories, and short rest breaks; that is all you can do.

It was unusual for all three of us to hit the wall at the same time, but it happened. The brutally hot weather hammered our bodies. There was not an ounce of shade to block the sun or offer even a momentary respite.

My mom was providing on-site assistance for us at the time, and she pulled her car off the side of the road and waved us over. We propped open the hatchback for shade and huddled under it. It wasn't much in the way of relief, but it was better than nothing.

"Just give it time," I told my guys. "No hurry."

We did our best to cool down by putting cold washcloths on our faces and drenching our hair with ice-cold water. A couple of minutes later, my brother Josh, who was all over the place getting video shots for the documentary, pulled up.

"What do you need?" he asked.

"You know what sounds good, brother? Popsicles."

"Sounds better than good," Tyler agreed with a smile.

"Popsicles it is," Josh said. "I'll see what I can find."

Josh took off, and we packed up Mom's car. We threw wet towels over our heads and started running again. Exactly a mile later, here came my brother to the rescue with fruit Popsicles from who knows where.

"You're a lifesaver," Hickey said to him.

Funny how little things can make a big difference. One fruit Popsicle pushed me out of my low moment and quickly turned it to a high one. I guess I needed sugar. I guess I also needed the distraction and the camaraderie. Once that icy treat was consumed, my legs generated some much-needed liveliness. I regained my mental energy and started to run strong. So strong that I dropped

Tyler and Josh. I didn't mean to, but I felt good and took advantage of my momentum.

The plan was to stop for lunch at mile thirty, which was going to be Tyler's end point. I ran right by it. I had found my best running pace of the entire two days and wanted to use this sudden burst to my advantage. The bad news was that I did not get to say goodbye to Tyler. He had given the Limitless run thirty good miles and I could not have been more appreciative of his support.

My "runner's high" carried me to mile thirty-four before my need for fuel prompted me to stop. Our two RVs made their way up the Edison Highway, and they had our aid station up and running in minutes. We were parked next to an orange grove on the outskirts of Bakersfield, which meant the only shade we had came from the RVs. It didn't matter. We were halfway through Day 2, we were eating a very tasty lunch, and everyone was in good spirits.

I looked around me. Stephanie, JoJo, my mom and brother, my great friends. So much support and love. Everyone on our crew was pushing and sacrificing for this one mission. It was not just about the guys doing the running. I could never have considered the Limitless project without a great support team, much less made it happen. These were all men and women (and kids) who believed in what we were trying to accomplish as much as I did.

I believe in "attitudinal contagion," meaning the attitude of the people around you will have a direct effect on your own personal attitude. I needed to surround myself with motivating, inspiring, and positive folks on this journey, and every single person on our crew exemplified those traits. It made for a "winning" team. We were all committed to this mission together. We were all pushing our limits. We all wanted to achieve a goal that many said could not be achieved. Best of all, we enjoyed each other's company, which made chasing that goal so much more enjoyable.

After a delicious grilled ham-and-cheese sandwich, I closed my eyes for two minutes. Two minutes of inward thinking and slow, deep breathing. I looked over at Josh, and he gave me a thumb's up. We clamored to our feet. I kissed my wife and daughter, and we continued along Edison Highway. We knew the desolate and boring roads would quickly change to mountains and soon we would be hammering up the hills of Tehachapi.

At this point, my body was beginning to stiffen up like a board. I am a positive guy and I generally find a way to focus on the positives. But as we hit the one-hundred-mile mark of our journey, I started to experience miniature specs of depression; I had so much running still ahead that it was hard not to feel the weight of the rather insane goal I had set. I was determined to push forward, but my body was fast becoming the culprit standing in the way of this effort.

From the orange grove, Hickey and I started with a few yards of walking, which quickly turned into our ultra-pace. A few miles down the road we were interrupted by a sign in the road that read: "No thru traffic." There were signs of construction, but the road looked accessible. We asked a couple of guys in work trucks what the situation was and decided, based on what we heard, to keep running. We told Stephanie and Lee (who was driving the other RV) to return to Highway 58 and meet us on the backside of Edison Highway. My mom, ever the rebel, would have none of it. She decided to stay with us no matter what the road conditions were. No, we weren't entirely convinced that cars could go through at this point, but we took the risk nonetheless.

A half mile farther on, we literally ran head-on into a deserted road construction zone. The paved road turned to dirt, but we could see where the paving resumed some ways ahead. We kept moving. Mom followed, weaving her way through the dusty and disassembled road like an off-road warrior. Thank God she did, because we absolutely needed every cube of ice and ounce of water she was providing us.

As we looked up the road ahead, the rolling hills seemed never-ending. This was a classic moment. The transformation of road conditions seemed to ignite our mental energy. Running on the flat and tedious roads of Bakersfield was behind us, and we were eager for new terrain. The conditions were not what some would call ideal. The temperature hovered in the mid-90s and the hills were taxing, but both Hickey and I seemed to gain strength as we began the trek up the hills.

Back home, we are fortunate to have access to some of the best running roads in the area. A short, fifteen-mile drive from my house is one of our favorites: Yokohl Valley. "Yokohl" is a small rural countryside that guides you through undulating landscapes of horse pastures, country living, and stunning beauty. Given the rolling hills, steep mountain climbs, and peaceful environment, it is a prime spot for training. I have done everything from hill repeats, to long bike rides, to long runs up in Yokohl Valley. One of my favorite workouts is called the "Oak Tree" repeats. Oak Tree is a popular destination for runners and bikers. It acts as a natural pit stop, where athletes take the time to enjoy the views of Yokohl Valley, talk with friends, and eat a snack before continuing along. "Oak Tree" repeats take place on the one-mile ascent up to the Oak Tree. The climb averages a six- to eight-percent incline. When completed eight or ten consecutive times, it makes for a challenging training session.

Another classic training site is the epic Rocky Hill in Exeter. Exeter is a small city located just ten miles east of Visalia. Rocky Hill is a one-mile climb, averaging a five- to eight-percent gradient and is a hot spot for local runners, cyclists, and triathletes. In preparation for Limitless, I would work this one-mile hill over and over for two hours. I would climb up Rocky Hill, reach the top, turn around, run back down, and repeat this cycle for two hours.

Oak Tree and Rocky Hill were the type of workouts I put together to gain strength on hills just like the ones we were facing now, and they were paying dividends.

Running with Hickey always has a positive affect on me. When we're together, I sometimes feel this sudden urge to pick up my pace. It's not that I'm trying to drop him—it's not that at all—it's all about pushing us to run a little faster. I suspect he does the same to me.

This was exactly what happened once we hit the hills beyond Bakersfield. No one got dropped, but there we were, pushing our bodies to the limit, almost as if we were in a race. This would be one hell of a climb in even the best of conditions, but this being mile 110 of our trek and with temperatures in the 90s, it made the run that much more punishing.

Despite that, it was a moment to be cherished. We were singing, laughing, and chatting about things that had nothing whatsoever to do with Limitless.

As we charged up the hill, a song my dad had written popped into my head and I let loose, running and singing:

I'm gonna be a leader someday,
a leader someday,
a leader someday,
I'm gonna be a leader someday, yes I am.
I'm gonna be like George Washington,
George Washington,
George Washington,
I'm gonna be like George Washington, yes I am.
I'm gonna be like Jim Barnes,
Jim Barnes,
Jim Barnes,

I'm gonna be like Jim Barnes, yes I am!

I'm not sure how much Jim appreciated the song, but Hickey and I had a helluva time singing it.

There were times when silence fell, and we listened to the clatter of our footsteps on the pavement. No cars on the road, no birds chirping, no words of advice or counsel from our traveling bicycle companion. Just a couple guys running; it made for peaceful moments.

Yeah, these hills made for a new change of pace and some memorable scenery, but they also beat us up pretty hard. We walked periodically to renew our energy, but the key was to keep moving forward. My brother Josh and his cameraman Dave caught up with us as we were hiking up a particularly precipitous hill. They rarely stopped shooting footage, but this time they had cold Gatorade and snacks to share, so we stopped for a few minutes, sat on the tailgate of their truck, and refueled. I asked my brother how much longer we had to climb. He said, "A few miles." Loved that answer.

We kept going.

One step at a time, one breathe at a time, Hickey and I would eventually fight off every hill and reach the summit of the mountain. You have no idea how relieved we were to see the RVs parked in a nice shady area awaiting our arrival. Stephanie, Lee, and the crew had literally set up our rest stop in the middle of the road since they knew it was closed to traffic.

Stephanie and my mom had chairs arranged around a card table. They had food and cold drinks laid out for us and an unspoken message: it was time to rest. "Thank God."

Spirits were high. The music was blaring. Hickey and I were lying down with our feet in ice. Jim was up dancing, his Cheshire smile wide with mischief. JoJo and her mom were making up their own dance steps. Mom, Lee, and the rest of the crew were laughing and tapping their feet.

All I could do was smile. True, I was pretty hammered at this stage of the run. My feet were swollen, my legs were smashed, and my mind was in a fog of fatigue, amazement, and sheer exhaustion. Lying down for fifteen minutes was the next best thing to sex with my beautiful wife, but I knew we needed to get up, get motivated, and keep running. It was a gloomy thought, knowing we still had twenty-something miles yet to run that day.

Within minutes, we came to another crossroad in our route. The only way to get to the Woodland-Tehachapi Road (which directed us to Tehachapi, our next stop for the night) was via Highway 58. We couldn't run it because it was illegal walking, running, or otherwise being on foot on highways or freeways as busy as 58. We didn't have much choice. Hickey and I hitched a ride in one of the RVs and drove east on Highway 58 for six miles to the Woodland-Tehachapi Road.

One part of me didn't like the decision, but it actually gave me a chance to rest, change into fresh clothes, and get my mindset ready for the evening ahead. It would be another long night of running, so this short rest helped rejuvenate both my body and mind.

After a change of clothes and some much-needed calories, I exited the RV ready to run. This was the first time in two days that I would be running solo. This was the first time when I would be without a pace runner. Hickey had seen me through the day, and now I was on my own. Just me, Jim, and his trusty bike.

I don't know if it's obvious, but I love being around people. It is what I live for. Positive relationships are what make the world go around, at least my world. But sometimes a person thrives in a moment of solitude, and this was one of them. Jim was close at hand, but he rode in silence, allowing me to run in quiet. I really enjoyed the isolation and took full advantage of it. I got inside my head, listened to my thoughts, and regained some emotional energy. It had been a long two days, and I needed some stillness at this point. The running was tasking my physical energy. It was also tasking my emotional and mental energy. This was a good time to just allow everything to soak in, zone out, and prepare for the upcoming miles.

Running the Woodland-Tehachapi Road was like a soothing period of meditation. The sun was starting to set, the mountains were reflecting its golden light, and my footsteps fell into a soothing cadence. It was another perfect moment.

While I'm good at enjoying moments like this, I am also fearful of them. I know full well that there is always an end to "perfect" times. The end scares the shit out of me. A very real part of me wishes that these "perfect" situations would last forever. Another more realistic part of me knows that they never do, and we move on. Life moves on.

Here I was, running in company with a gorgeous sunset, and myriad thoughts rumbled through my head:

My wedding night. Flawless. I was marrying the perfect woman. Our friends and family, the people we cared about the most, were there to celebrate with us. The entire night was magical. It was a great party, a wonderful celebration of love, and the launch of a new life ahead. Of course, the night eventually ended and became a wonderful memory.

Such is the nature of life, and, of course, there are so many of these situations. I must admit, however, that I live for them. I love having a good time with the most important people in my life. However, these times also scare me. I know how short-lived many of these great moments are. Life moves fast, really fast. That is what fuels my motivation to live so hard every day of my life. I want to make the best of every situation. I want to find the positives. I want to leave every experience knowing I did my best. But this persistent hard living also tires me out. I get overwhelmed. I spread myself way to thin. My emotional energy gets zapped. I am constantly try-ing to find the balance in my life. I'm constantly . . .

"Stop, Justin," I said out loud. "Just run, man. Just run."

So I did. After soloing for five miles, my brother Josh decided to join me. How cool was that. Josh, by his own admission, is in average shape. He is definitely not an experienced runner. But here he was. He must have noticed that I needed someone out there with me. How incredibly honorable was that for him to step up and run with me, two brothers side by side.

He was dressed in his khaki cargo shorts, a cotton T-shirt, cotton socks, and his casual New Balance shoes. Oh, and he was going commando! A serious faux pas in the running world. Why? One word: chaffing. Chaffing can literally stop a runner in his or her tracks. But that's Josh for you. My bro. His motivation was sparked and he was ready to go. I was happy to have him by my side, climbing the hills heading into Tehachapi with the sun set-ting right before our eyes. We chatted. We laughed. We analyzed the whole situation.

Naturally, it didn't take Josh long to get philosophical.

"Man, this is crazy, dude. I can't believe you're doing this." See? Pretty philosophical. And then the inevitable, "How're you feeling?"

"I'm good, man," I replied, though I know I sounded a trifle annoyed.

I didn't elaborate or say much else because I was battling the onset of a low spot; the hills around Tehachapi will do that to you.

When these low spots hit, I just needed to put my head down and run. Stay focused. Blanket my mind. As nicely as I could, I would tell whomever I was running with, "I need some silence right now."

Of course, this silence didn't last long. Something would usu-ally pop into my head, and I would have to share it. And if it wasn't me, it was Jim. The guy had a thousand stories to tell, and when his memory dredged one up, he told it. Right there on the spot. I didn't mind. It almost always helped me slip back into a "runner's high." Jim knew this too, of course.

It was quite the scene climbing the switchback roads up into the Tehachapi hills. The sun vanished and we were now running in the pitch black of night. The road was narrow, the stars were bright, and the night was calm. Running this particular road was dangerous. There was no shoulder. Josh and I were in the middle of the road. Mom was in her car some lengths behind with the headlights beaming. This helped keep cars in check if they were coming up on us too fast. Luckily, there was a minimum amount of traffic, and what there was didn't seem to be in a big hurry.

We would stop every three or four miles so I could rest, hydrate, and collect my thoughts. These small breaks would rejuvenate me so I could pump out another three- or four-mile spurt. One spurt after another. *Just keep moving, Justin. You got this.*

Physically, I was worn out. Mentally, I was like a yo-yo, up and down. There was only one solution. I battled the lows and found great appreciation from the highs.

I was actually running quite strongly. My body seemed to respond to the hills. It was probably my diminutive frame that enabled me to drive up the mountains. Or maybe it was because I was always training on hills. Or maybe it was the caffeine from the Mountain Dew I was drinking. Whatever the reason, I didn't mind the increased strength required in the mountains.

I was impressed that my brother was able to stay with my pace. I didn't know how long it would last, but it didn't matter. He was with me now and doing well. I was grateful. I enjoyed the camaraderie.

Getting to the top of the Woodland-Tehachapi Road was a watershed moment; I knew we were close to concluding this massive day of running and it couldn't come too soon.

We had decided to headquarter in an RV park that Lee had found on the outskirts of town, but that meant I still had six miles to run. Six miles is not a big run, but this last stretch through Tehachapi was tough. I was battling every footstep, every stride. We were hitting the 130-mile mark for the entire trip. I was tired, hungry, and desperate for sleep.

As much as I tried avoiding the thought that I still had 170 miles to go, I couldn't fight it off. Talk about a glum feeling.

It was 10:00 as my snail's pace inched me through the city of Tehachapi. I just wanted to find the RV Park and be done with it.

I had two miles to go when a wave of annoyance and frustration swept over me. I slowed to a walk just to keep moving. The annoyance signaled a drop in blood sugar and a need for food. My saving grace was a Burger King up ahead. I called to Rocky and asked him if he could grab me an order of French fries. That's how desperate I was. On the other hand, you have never seen an order of fries devoured so quickly and so thoroughly.

That and the sight of my brother refusing to stop, limping along and determined to finish the night with me, gave me a jolt of positive energy. He said his knee was a little sore, but he wasn't going to let that stop him. I was inspired. He'd been with me for ten miles. For someone who does not run on a regular basis, ten miles is a very arduous run and I was impressed.

We turned a last corner, and the RV park reared up to meet us. What a sight! After another day of running sixty-plus miles, to say I was relieved to call it a night would be a gross understatement. Knowing I had still had six-and-a-half marathons left to go was cause for a wave of depression, but I was determined not to let this emotion show. Like I do with many of my emotions, I kept it to myself. Not sure why, exactly. Maybe I do not like feeling vulnerable. Maybe it is because I like to be in control. I know I should learn to open up and express my feelings and emotions more freely. Selfishly, doing so relieves stress. The run was helping with this. If I needed help, I asked. If I was feeling down, I told people. If I needed to cry, I did. I also realized that to live a positive and meaningful life, I needed supportive and trustworthy people in my corner, people who were both empathetic and sympathetic. Fortunately, I had exactly those kinds of people in my life.

I flopped into the nearest chair. I devoured two Burger King hamburgers and another large order of fries. I drank water and Gatorade. I was not surprised that my body was breaking down. Two days of running all day had definitely taken its toll.

Rocky asked me how I was doing. I sarcastically answered, "I just ran 130 miles in two days, so I guess I'd say I'm a little tired."

He knew that I was pretty beat up. I was not smiling much that night. I just wanted to close my eyes, lie down, and rest my body, but I let Rocky stretch me out to relieve my muscles. It helped.

I took a quick RV shower, put on some fresh clothes, and headed to bed. Another long day of running was in my future.

I went to bed thinking, *Tomorrow morning it's going to be hard as hell to get out of bed, so prepare yourself.*

Day 2: 60 miles

Total: 127 miles

CHAPTER 14

....

IT'S STARTING TO GET HARD

Day 3, Tehachapi—Angeles National Forest

The RV park was not the best place to sleep after running 127 miles in a two-day span. First, the trains roaring past the park were unbearably loud. Second, the bed in the RV was not particularly comfortable. Third, and most important, sleeping with a two-year-old (who essentially owned the bed), is not conducive to deep and rejuvenating sleep.

I felt my burning muscles and sore joints every time I moved. On the other hand, some sleep was better than none at all.

Our goal for Day 3 was seventy miles. We wanted to start by 5:45 a.m. so we could get some miles in before the sun came up. When my eyes snapped open at 5:25, I was completely down in the dumps. I still had six and a half marathons to run, and it was a tough thought for my mind to grasp.

My body was achy as I rolled out of bed and started to move around. I did not have any major issues going on, however, such as knee or back pain. Overall I was just physically and mentally wiped out. I did my normal morning routine. I ate breakfast, Rocky stretched me out, and we prepared our gear for the day ahead. We all huddled together as Jim delivered the morning's spiritual message. Having Jim with us on this adventure was like having our very own guiding angel; it was such a gift. I get emotional thinking back on his Limitless presence. Here is a man in his mid-60s, a retired schoolteacher, a man full of life, who had willingly and enthusiastically committed to a project of this magnitude. It was as if Jim was put on the Earth to guide and support other people to better living. He was our spiritual guide, and we could not have done it without him.

As my body was breaking down and my mind was in full battle mode, Jim's morning prayer softened my anguish and gave me a sense of tranquility. It gave me the wherewithal to think about the day ahead without panicking. It was going to be a grueling day running straight into the Mojave Desert and eventually entering the Angeles Forest. I did my best to keep things positive.

One step at a time. Just keep going, I thought.

We finished our group huddle and blessed the day ahead. It was time to run.

As Hickey and Jim were finishing their preparations, I set out alone; the three of us would meet up a few miles down the road, while my mom and dad drove support, fifty yards or so behind me.

The morning was dark and cold so I started with arm warmers and a wind vest. I was glad to be alone those first two miles, because I was hit with a serious wave of emotion and started crying. These were not easy tears tinseling my cheeks; I was balling like a baby. It was difficult to fathom that I would be running seventy miles today after already putting in 127 miles in forty-eight hours. Simply put, the lows were getting lower. It was a miserable feeling.

I now started to encounter the unknowns of ultra-running. I was pushing through my physical limits. My body would be hurting the rest of the trip; there was no way around that. *Get use to it, Justin.* My mind, spirit, and determination needed to carry me forward. All I wanted was to drive forward and push out of the hole.

I did my best to put one foot in front of the other. After about thirty minutes of slow and depressed running, somehow my despondent emotions turned into positive strength. My legs loosened up and started to feel strong. My mind suddenly felt fresh and motivated. It was a complete 180-degree turnaround. These first few miles reinforced a valuable lesson for me. When an obstacle or a tough time smacks you in the face, keep pushing and driving forward. Quitting is not an option. Building resilience and constructing a "get back up" attitude is highly critical to withstand the harshness life produces. With continued persistence, we can chisel our way through those obstacles and strength will be gained. You have to fight through the tough times in life. You have to battle those uncomfortable moments that nobody wants to encounter. In my case, I had to keep running. No other choice.

I stopped at a gas station to use the restroom, and Jim and Hickey were there waiting for me. We pressed on together, Jim on his trusty bike, Hickey running by my side. We had high spirits in concert with the rising sun. The power of the sun was unrivalled. It gave us a "new beginning" to a fresh day. At least this was our philosophical metaphor. The Tehachapi Mountains were past us and we were running right into the heart and soul of the desert.

We turned and headed south on Tehachapi Willow Springs Road. This road, at sunrise, was desolate, quiet, and peaceful. Wind fans were sprawled throughout this golden land, and it was a picturesque scene as they circled clockwise. We were directly west of the Mojave Desert. The morning air was crisp and cool, very good for running. Hickey and I were excited, knowing our good friend Landon Brokaw would be joining us this morning. A fresh mind and equally fresh legs were always something to look forward to in an ultra-run environment, so we were anxious for Landon's arrival.

After my emotional start this morning, I got into a groove, and the first half-marathon flew by. Positive conversation assisted our migration south. Fifteen miles into the day, we saw Landon parked at a rest stop. He was raring to go and fell into lockstep. Landon's longest run to date was fourteen miles. Today, his goal was to run a full marathon with us—twenty-six miles—but I didn't want him feeling any undue pressure. Just like I told all of our pace runners, I said, "Just take it one step at a time, Landon. Manage your nutrition, accept the pace we're running, and just keep moving forward."

Easier said than done sometimes.

The plan was for Mom to drop Dad at the rest stop, where he would slide behind the wheel of Landon's car and drive support for us over the next few hours.

What can I say about my mom and dad? They had my back during the entire Limitless project, and here they were driving support mile after mile. I could not have done it without them. Something I can say about a lot of people.

Hickey, Landon, and I ran together for a mile or so before we took a quick break to eat some food.

"What the hell? Look at this setup," Landon said when he saw our aid station all prepped and ready for our arrival. Seeing the look on our pace runners' faces was always amusing to me. I'm not sure what they were expecting, but it was probably not the well-oiled machine they got. I would sit down, food in my hand, and Rocky would begin working on my feet. It was like a pit crew at the Indy 500.

At this aid station, we ate chicken noodle soup. This is a common food in the ultra-running world. With the amount of sweating we were doing, our sodium levels were depleted, and the soup was a good source of sodium and calories. It was also soothing on the stomach and easy to digest.

I was in good spirits. Having Landon in the fold was uplifting. Seeing my wife and daughter was uplifting. Listening to Lee and Rocky badgering each other was uplifting. Hearing Jim humming some unknown tune was uplifting.

I was up and on my feet again after a short fifteen-minute break and ready to move forward. We filled our water bottles and took off.

As we hit the long, straight roads of the desert, we could tell it was going to be the hottest day we'd experienced so far. And when I say, "long and straight roads," that is exactly what they were. They seemed endless. I looked toward the horizon, and all I could see was a road that kept going. (Talk about Limitless.) The "one step at a time" mindset was all we had to rely on.

By 11:00 a.m., we were already feeling the cooked pavement as it radiated heat straight through our bodies. Hot sun, hot desert roads, and not a speck of shade equated to tough running conditions. We trudged through the desert lands, running at a slow ultra-pace, but we kept moving forward, one step at time.

In the middle of the barren desert, I hit the 150-mile mark. I had reached the halfway point. I had just run 150 miles in two and a half days. We stopped at a corner store—probably the only store within ten miles—and Stephanie bought a bottle of wine as a celebratory symbol of our journey thus far. We took a short fluid break (no, I didn't drink any wine; that would have to wait) just to collect ourselves, cool down, and rest the legs. Most people would be pretty ecstatic after running 150 miles. I was subdued and knew plenty of work was yet to be done.

Shortly, we would be meeting up with our next pace runner, my good friend Lindsey Clemens. Lindsey is an awesome endurance athlete and her presence was much needed at this point of the run. Her positive energy is contagious, and we were excited to have her aboard. Plus, we would now be a group of four running together, and there was no way that couldn't boost my spirits in the most positive way.

Hickey, Landon, and I had been at it for several miles when we heard a car approaching from behind. We heard someone tapping their horn, and then we heard Lindsey calling our names. She pulled up alongside us and leaned out the window. "I don't suppose you boys are in need of a lift," she said with a wide smile.

"A lift, no. Company, absolutely," I answered.

"Join us, girl. The weather is perfect," Jim called, waving at the scorching sun.

"Our crew is a couple of miles up the road," I told her.

"Meet you there."

By the time we reached our RVs, Lindsey was suited up and ready to roll. We fueled up, refilled our water bottles, and set out again.

There we were, Hickey, Landon, Lindsey, and I, running the desert roads at a steady, ultra-run clip. And of course, Jim was on his trusty bike keeping us thoroughly entertained. It was a like scene from a movie. Well, it was a scene from a movie. Josh and his crew were out there getting as much footage for the documentary as they could. They seemed to have a camera in my face the entire run. I didn't mind, though. I just did my thing and pretended the camera wasn't there.

Part of doing my thing was yo-yoing between positive and negative thoughts; the desert did that to you. When a wave of negativity hit, I just dropped my hat low, got inside my brain, and push forward. I listened to the voices of my fellow runners. Listened to their conversations, their laughter, their stories. Their stories, gratefully, gave me something to ponder other than my own pain. Most of the time when I go out for a run, I'm comfortable being by myself. It's my time to be alone, get away from the busyness and business of life, and zone out. On the other hand, I definitely enjoy the company of a small group of extremely driven and positive runners. The environment lifts you up, even when you might be feeling like roadkill.

Thanks goodness for their company.

Our next goal was the town of Lancaster. This would be Landon's stopping point. From there, we planned to go south to Palmdale. Because I had Lindsey and Landon pacing me, Hickey decided to rest up and catch a ride with one of the RVs. It was a good decision. He needed the break, and I would need his presence once we entered the Angeles Forest.

While the heat was zapping my energy, the companionship of Lindsey and Landon created a surge of energy. We trotted into Lancaster, and all I could feel was a wave of appreciation for the support Landon had shown us. He had run thirty-one miles! A personal best. Talk about Limitless.

At the beginning, I don't think I knew how important my pace runners would be in this endeavor. But as they would peel off one by one, I would say my goodbyes, express my heartfelt gratitude, and then it was back to the grind. I had more work to do. I owed it to them and everyone else on our amazing crew to make the most of their efforts. It gave me an extra nudge, and I needed all the nudges I could get.

Lancaster was also break time. I needed food. I needed to get my feet up. I needed to hug my daughter. My feet seemed to be getting more swollen all the time, but it was nothing that impeded my running, at least not at the time. It seemed to be at its worst when I stopped, and the blood rushed to my feet.

I ate my favorite grilled ham-and-cheese sandwich, drank some fluids under Rocky's watchful eye, and shut my eyes. After that, I soaked my feet in ice water for five minutes, and Rocky worked on them to promote blood flow. Thank goodness for his patience and his professionalism; I'm not sure I could have massaged feet as beat up, sweaty, and dirty as mine, but Rocky never wavered.

Lindsey and I set out a few minutes later, and let me tell you, she was running solid. She just tucked in next to me like an "angel," giving me wings and nudging me ever closer to my goal.

We headed west until we hit the Sierra Highway. The Sierra would take us south to Palmdale and eventually into the epic mountains of the Angeles National Forest.

An hour outside of Lancaster, I ran head-first into yet another wall. First came the silence; then came a wave of annoyance. My mood sank, and I was ambushed by an unexpected need for food. All told, I just needed to get off my feet for a few minutes, so we found a patch of grass near a shopping center and sat down. It must have been an unusual site seeing "a couple of runners" just hanging out on some random grassy knoll. I wasn't worried about appearances at that point. I scarfed down an avocado burrito, drank some coffee, and just chilled.

I was experiencing an interesting phenomenon. My hunger was seemingly impossible to satisfy. I would eat, I would feel relatively full for a few miles, and then starvation would lay waste to me in a matter of just a few minutes. It was tough to manage, but we did the best we could.

In this case, we clocked a five-minute break, got up, and ran another twenty minutes. We found the RVs parked in the dilapidated lot of a local school. It was like coming across the most irresistible mirage in the world. I just needed to sit down for a few minutes. I needed to eat again and close my eyes.

Weary and depleted: those were the only two words I could think of to describe how my body was feeling.

We had a full posse with us. Josh Hickey's wife, Jaime, my sister-in-law Kimmie, and our good friend Kelsey had arrived, and they jumped right into the adventure. It was good to see everyone's smiling faces. The support was humbling. Hickey was in good spirits and encouraged me to consume calories. He was right; I needed every calorie I could get.

Hickey joined back with us, and I appreciated his company. Lindsey was still running right by my side, "carrying" me. Jim was on his bike, giving me water and food any time I asked for it and stories when I didn't. These people were my saviors.

We would need to run a couple more miles before we hit the Sierra Highway. This made for a positive feeling because we would soon be headed south. Heading south meant that we were moving toward Los Angeles, which would be our final destination. It felt good. Once we hit the Sierra Highway, there was a bike lane that proved to be a Godsend. For once, we could just run without the worry of traffic. Nice and peaceful. But right when we hit this bike trail, I fell into a rather deep hole. These low spots would just arise with no warning. What's more, they seemed to be coming and going with greater frequency. My mood would become subdued, my head would go down, and I would just get inside my head. Nothing specifically would trigger these low spots. The ups and downs of ultra-running, I guess. I also viewed it as a metaphor for life. We all experience low spots. We all experience tragedy. Whether it's related to our profession or our personal lives, the key is to find strength and determination to battle back. *Put your head down, put one foot in front of the other, and keep moving forward.* The low spot will eventually subside. I was proof positive of this.

As I was battling inside my head, my sister-in-law Kimmie jumped out of one of our support cars all decked out in her gear and started running with us. I think I said something nonchalant like, "Hey, Kimmie, thanks for joining us," but what I remember most was the boost it gave me.

It was so cool when "non-runners" joined our group, even for a short time. The deeper we were getting into this massive run, the more elevated the human spirit became. Yes, the lows were depressive, but the strength of the human spirit always seemed to triumph. The positive energy was contagious; it didn't just drive me, it seemed to affect everyone we came in contact with. Here was Kimmie, jumping in next to three people who ran for both exercise and competition, and she fit in perfectly, her energy giving us all a boost.

Kimmie didn't say much as she ran. She just stayed at my shoulder, reminding me that support does not have to be "loud." Support can sit quietly in the shadows and play a tremendously vital role. I knew Kimmie was there. That was all that mattered. Hickey and Lindsey felt the same thing; here was another set of broad shoulders to propel us forward.

As for me? I was just grateful for anyone willing to put in a few miles with me. It made the whole experience so much better. It inspired me. It drove me. It sparked a very real sense of responsibility.

I didn't even see the local television reporter standing right in the middle of the bike path. Hickey said, "Justin, we have company. Looks like the local news."

I looked up. She had her camera set up and was apparently getting some footage as we came her way. I stopped. "Hey, how are you?" I managed to say.

"I'm good. Can I ask a few questions?" she said after introducing herself.

I have to admit that I was a little hesitant. Not out of shyness. Not me. I'm not the shy type. I hesitated because I was in such a low stop on the run. Then I thought: *What the hell. Maybe this will help.* Plus, we had spent so much time and energy promoting Limitless over the last few months, and here was a reporter anxious to spread the Limitless story. She asked how far we had progressed and what our next steps were. She asked how I was feeling and how our crew was holding up. She asked if I expected to make it. "Three hundred miles in one hundred hours? That's an amazing goal."

"We're giving it everything we have," I replied. "I would love to have you at the finish line when we get there."

We talked for another couple of minutes, and I was surprised how much the interview actually lifted my spirits. I was surprised how much my mood had improved when it was over. I went from a quiet and passive state to my normal happy-go-lucky self.

After she had packed up her camera and headed back to town, we laughed about the stories we had shared and spent a couple minutes watching the sunset. It turned out to be the perfect break in the day, the perfect way to break a down cycle.

We continued on. The bike path stretched out before us. The sun continued to set to our right, a bright palette of yellow, orange, and pink painting the sky. We entered the city of Palmdale and marked the 175-mile-mark in our journey. We had been running since 5:45 a.m. We still had roughly fifteen miles before we hit the rolling hills of the Angeles National Forest, our goal at night's end. The bike trail led us south. It was time for a dinner break. I was hungry! Everyone was hungry.

We stopped in a parking lot fronting a local business complex. The RVs were already there, with food and drinks laid out. To my great surprise, there were two local Visalians waiting for us as well. Raul Gonzalez was the founder of a local group in town called the Maverick Runners. Antonio Luevano worked at the local shoe store, Sole2Soul Sports.

"We thought you'd like some company," Raul said, throwing his arms around us.

"You're kidding. You going to run with us?" I said.

"That's why we're here, amigo," Antonio said with a grin.

My spirits immediately elevated. These two guys had come all the way out here to see us to the end of our night. I am not going to lie: we needed the support. It had been a helluva day. I could not have asked for a more experienced runner than Raul. He had extensive experience in the ultra-distance world and had completed numerous ultra-distance marathons. His knowledge and familiarity of ultra-distance running was a major plus at this point.

My first priority after welcoming Raul and Antonio into the fold was fuel, whatever satisfied my hunger and kept my stomach at ease. Top Ramen and soda seemed to do the trick at this aid station. I changed my clothes, stretched, and set off again to the cheers of our support team.

We had some of the best runners around pushing the pace toward the Angeles Forest: Lindsey, Raul, Hickey, Antonio, Kimmie, and me. I was stoked. The adrenaline was flowing. My legs felt strong. We lost Hickey a mile in when he decided not to push the pace we were setting and decided to rejoin us again when we hit the hills.

The five of us ran straight through Palmdale. Sierra Highway turned right onto the Angeles Forest Highway and the running became immediately precarious. Similar to Highway 65 on Day 1, the cars flashing past seemed to be attracted to our headlamps and reflectors. Raul ran out in front of us a number of paces to warn the cars away from the limited shoulder we were running on. Essentially we were running on the fog line and spending far too much energy watching out for speeding cars.

"Car up!" we yelled over and over again. Delirium set in. I guess I shouldn't have been surprised after seventy-two hours of running. All I can say in retrospect is how very grateful I was for my pace runners and their attention to safety during this hectic part of the run. It wasn't much fun.

These miles were a constant battle. One foot in front of the other. It doesn't sound like much of a mantra, but it was all I had. It was now close to 8:00 p.m. My body and mind were completely spent and all I had was my physical and mental autopilot and a strong and seemingly indefatigable sense of spirit.

We wanted to get as close to the two-hundred-mile marker that night as possible. That was our goal. That was our war cry.

We took a rest stop right before heading into the brutal and challenging hills of the Angeles National Forest. I collected my thoughts, talked myself into some positive thinking, and consumed a Power Bar gel, a quick energy fix. We rested for ten minutes, which was probably eight minutes too many, because I could hardly get out of my chair.

"Take it slow, hombre," Raul said encouragingly. "Let's walk a bit to get the wheels moving again."

I didn't walk. I staggered. Literally. Staggering eventually turned into a slow shuffle. By some miracle, this slow shuffle morphed into a slow jog.

By the time we started the trek up the hills, I was more or less back in the groove. Raul and Antonio were solid pace runners. I couldn't have asked for better. Raul and Hickey—who had rejoined us at our rest stop—hammered up the hills, which kept me on pace, more or less. We needed Hickey now. The forest roads were sketchy, and his experience was priceless. Lindsey was just up ahead and nothing short of amazing. She was beyond the marathon distance for the day and was still going strong. Kimmie continued to be an inspiration, consistently driving up the hills and exuding extraordinarily positive energy. She was embarking on a twelve-mile run, which would be the longest run in her life. Here I was, at the back of the pack trudging up the mountain with Antonio running right next to me and doing his best to keep me company. My drive and determination were strong, but my body and mind were past depleted.

These hills put the exclamation point on Day 3. I wanted Limitless, I got it. Nothing like climbing six- to eight-percent gradient hills at the end of a seventy-mile day. I would have to walk sections to just keep moving forward, but I did. The plan was to find a spot along the Angeles Forest Highway to set up camp and call it a night. The crew's first choice was too close to the highway, so we kept running. At that moment, I felt pretty good; why not find a spot where we would be more comfortable for the night? So we pressed on.

It was now close to 10:30 p.m. Here we were, six runners on a mission, climbing through the Angeles National Forest, living life to the fullest. It was an unforgettable moment.

After feeling a burst of strength for a few minutes, I started hitting the wall for the umpteenth number of times. *Here we go again*, I thought. I actually bonked pretty hard. My body was in full revolt. I was also starving and ready to eat dinner.

"How much farther to camp?" I heard myself ask.

Someone—I'm not sure who—called back, "One or two miles, Justin. Keep moving. You got it."

One or two miles. Ok, I was good with that.

As it turned out, we ended up running for thirty more minutes. Either I was running very slowly or there were actually three or four miles left, not one or two. You never tell a runner they have fewer miles than they really do. This unintentional oversight really pissed me off. For the first time, I let my frustration get the best of me. Rocky came up next to me, and I made sure to let him know how I was feeling. "Rocky, from now on, do not tell us we have one or two miles left when really we really have three or four."

He just nodded his head and said, "You got it. I'll check it out. You're doing great, man. Sorry about the miscommunication."

As I walked up one of the final hills, I munched on a Payday bar that Jim had in his bag. Boy, was this the spark of energy I needed to finish the night. And just as I was finishing the bar, Rocky came back down the hill and yelled out, "One more mile, guys! We're parked at the top of this next hill."

At this point, I took off and started racing up the hill. My reasoning was simple: the faster I ran, the faster I would be done for the night. I surged passed Antonio, then Kimmie, and finally Lindsey, Raul, and Hickey. I got a cheer or two out of them as I passed, and that certainly helped.

I finally reached the top of the hill and saw the RVs. They were parked side-by-side in a turnoff well off the road. The relief I felt was more than I can describe, like a breath of cool air lifting me up and carrying me home.

I had logged sixty-seven miles. Overall, we were at mile 194.

I glanced over my shoulder and watched my fellow runners coming home. I was so happy for Lindsey. She finished the night running close to thirty-four miles, a career best.

Later, she would write:

Ran through Mojave desert mid-day to Angeles Forest late night with Justin Levine and the Limitless crew. It was an experience I will never forget! Witnessing a part of his three-hundred-mile journey was incredible and truly life changing. It was an honor to run next to him and encourage him for half a day. I was able to push through limits and boundaries I never thought possible, and I already can't wait to do it again! Thank you, Justin, for making me a stronger woman! I fell in love with running after my time on the road with you and your team.

Admirably, Kimmie finished running twelve miles. She was sore and beat up from her run, but mentally energized, realizing her achievement.

I was also so thankful for Raul and Antonio and their courageous efforts. Extraordinary. Unfortunately, they had to drive back home that night and be at work the next morning. Imagine that. They had come all this way just to be part of Limitless. I was humbled by their support, humbled by the support from all the runners who gladly and courageously paced me through the day.

I will forever have a special place in my heart for them: Landon, Lindsey, Raul, Antonio, and Kimmie. And of course, my man Josh Hickey. It would not have happened without him.

I was exhausted. I sat down, ate a big bowl of pasta, and loaded up on fluids. It is hard to put into words how sore and beat up my body was. I am not much of a complainer, but at mile 194, I was physically and mentally spent. Now that the running was done for the day, chills began coursing throughout my entire body. I had pushed my immune system to its extreme, and now it was fighting back. I told myself I just needed some rest. I just needed time to recover. But as I curled up in bed, I was bombarded by a single, almost paralyzing thought: "I have one-hundred-plus more miles to go."

Day 3: 67 miles
Total: 194 miles

CHAPTER 15

LOOK AT HOW FAR YOU HAVE COME

Day 4: Angeles National Forest—Glendale

Personal improvement is the spice of life. At least it is the spice of my life.

Personal improvement keeps me humble and respectful to my family, my friends, my colleagues, and myself. It holds me accountable. I am constantly trying to improve every area of my life. I believe that when I am strong, healthy, and vibrant, I can give more to others. I set goals and strive for them. My work ethic is relentless. I know what it's like to be uncomfortable, and I know feeling uncomfortable is a sign of growth.

Creating this personal philosophy has changed my life. My optimism and vigor persists each and every day. For me, life should be lived with extreme positive energy. Please don't mistake this for some perfect and fairytale animation. Setting goals and seeking the uncomfortable comes with a good amount of bumps in the road. Challenging times are part of the package. I wouldn't have it any other way.

I know this much, however: striving for personal growth translates unmistakably into better living.

Right in the middle of my Limitless run, I realized I was facing fears I may not have even realized existed and weaknesses that had never show themselves before. My limitations became so

133

visual. I felt physical distress beyond any I had ever encountered. My vulnerability was on display for all to see. I could expand or I could fold up my tent and go home. In other words, this had turned into a demonstration of personal growth far beyond just some run.

I was pushing every inch of my body and mind, almost to the extent of a breakdown. But with each step, with each stride, no matter the degree of my physical hurt, my strength and determination kept winning. I was willing to sacrifice my own body to illustrate how determination and obsessive desire can and will see us to our goals, no matter how unobtainable they may seem along the way. The run, at this point, was now becoming less of a physical encounter than it was a mental and spiritual episode. I was beyond physical soreness. All I could do was put that aside. It came down to a single question: how badly did I want to achieve the goal of running three hundred miles in one hundred hours? Was I willing to forfeit my own physicality, step into my own head, and battle my own demons? Would I be able to set aside my physical anguish in the quest to keep moving forward?

Day 4, and these were the internal thoughts that I woke up embracing.

I arose at 5:30 despite a plan everyone had embraced last night to sleep in a bit. I was able to manage four hours of solid sleep. I woke up sporting sore legs, swollen feet, an essentially deprived body, a tired mind, and eyes that resisted opening despite all the challenges of the day, or maybe because of all the challenges of the day.

We wanted to be on the road by 7:00 a.m. The thinking was that we would take our time to get ready. My arches screamed from a day running on uneven pavement. Rocky taped them up and made the issue manageable. Other than sore arches and the normal body aches that come with running nearly two hundred miles in three days, I didn't have any unusual pain. My physical body seemed to be holding up pretty well. Running for this extreme distance, you would think the knees would start to hurt, the back would ache, or the hips would be in pain. That was not the case. I have a durable body purely from a DNA standpoint. During training, I spend endless amounts of time working on my core and my overall functional strength. This area of fitness is a critical component to staying healthy and injury-free as an athlete. I emphasize a focus on strength, balance, and mobility with all the athletes I coach.

The time ticked by. I was stalling. Guilty as charged. I had 106 miles to run. Our initial goal was to be done by 10:00 the next morning. I just wanted to sit back and enjoy a cup or two of coffee. The problem was, I knew what needed doing, and my damn sense of determination was pushing hard.

We gathered around our spiritual leader for our morning prayer. It seemed my depressive and fatigued state was contagious, because the crew was clearly a bit more somber than previous mornings.

Once again, however, Jim's spiritual message gave us hope.

He looked around at the crew and said, "I just want to thank you, on behalf of all of us. We would not be standing here this morning, at this time, if it weren't for our support team. You think of us before you think of yourself. If even fifty percent of the world thought this way, we would be so much better off. The Limitless project is above and beyond even what Justin imagined or dreamed. The impact it is having on other people's lives is amazing. This is not just about one man's journey, but a testimony to living life to the fullest and the spirit of those willing to help without thought of glory or reward."

Jim knew the perfect words to soften our hearts and strengthen our minds. He knew that physically we were hitting our limits and that, in order for us to achieve this massive goal, we needed strong spirits. The morning's prayer put positive words into our hearts and gave me that much-needed push to get the day going.

No one really knew I'd taken off.

I didn't tell anyone. As soon as our morning prayer concluded, I turned toward the road and set out, my pace slow and methodical. I just needed to move. I knew once we got going I would be fine, but those first few miles were just plain painful.

Exactly as it had happened the previous morning, a wave of emotion hit me like a ton of bricks as I began trekking up that first hill. I had no control over these emotions. It was as if they had a mind of their own. One minute I would be running strong and feel good, and the next, depression would surface. This was the rollercoaster I would battle from here on out.

Okay, bring it on.

Immediately, we knew that the first section of the Angeles National Forest would be difficult. Climbing the four- to eight-percent-grade hills, battling the wind, and dodging traffic, the first few hours of running would challenge us. After running for about twenty minutes, Jim and Josh met up with me.

"There you are. We didn't know you had left," said Jim.

"I just needed to get going," I said.

We were together again, the three amigos. I recited the lyrics to Jim Morrison's song, "Riders on the Storm," but replaced "riders" with "runners." We were "Runners on the Storm." We had coined this phrase during our training in Pismo Beach. Anything to keep our minds positive and happy. When we chanted these lyrics, or any lyrics for that matter, we smiled and it would lift our spirits.

It was windy and chilly. Hickey wore a jacket with a tied-up hoodie to block the wind. I wore my Visalia Triathlon Club vest, arm warmers, and a trucker hat tilted low. The scenery in the Angeles National Forest was spectacular—shadowy peaks dotted with towering pines—but it was difficult to enjoy the landscape. The steep hills, my aching body, and my emotional distress made the first ten miles tough. I put my head down and tried my to get into a groove.

Kelsey Schulte, a new face, had joined us as a pace runner. She had recently moved from Missouri to California for an internship at California Fitness Academy. She moved in with my family one month before this adventure. Talk about jumping into the fire! Although she came into our life at a hectic time, she fit in well. Kelsey was now the Change Your Life Manager at California Fitness Academy and integral to the business. Although classified as a non-runner, she was motivated to run with me in the Angeles National Forest. Kelsey recounted her experience in her journal.

Friday morning I woke up at 6:30 a.m. after sleeping great in the car. Justin headed out at 7:00 a.m. He ventured through the mountains and windy roads of the Angeles Forest. He hit mile 200 around 10:00 a.m. From mile 200 to mile 207, I ran with him. I almost stopped twice, but Justin encouraged me to keep going. I ran most of it with him and his two brothers. I stopped around 11:15 a.m. This was huge for me! Jim is the cyclist that has been with Justin every step of the way. Josh and Dave have been filming nonstop. Stephanie and Lee are driving the RVs."

Everyone clapped and cheered when we made it to mile two hundred. I just waved, thanked them quietly, and kept running. I didn't want to celebrate, because I was struggling. I was doing my best to stay focused and keep moving forward. I was fixated on the one hundred miles ahead of me. I had just run two hundred miles! But I was too concerned about the upcoming mileage to appreciate my achievement. I looked ahead, focused on how much of the mountain we still had to hike. I didn't realize that I should have looked down the mountain to see how far we had come.

In life, we must value the journey we have taken to get to the present. Knowing where you have come from is just as important as knowing where you want to go. This was a huge life lesson for me.

As I was battling this tough start, a car pulled up next to me. I didn't immediately look over. *What is this car doing?* To my surprise, it was my older brother, Jason, who had driven down from Northern California. I was so surprised to see him.

"Are you going to run?" I asked.

"Yup, that's why I am here." He pulled over to the side of the road, got out, changed into his running shoes and started running with me. My dad took the wheel of his car. My spirits were immediately lifted. To have my older brother out there supporting me was special. Jason wasn't a serious runner; he had just been training to lose weight. His normal training runs were only four to eight miles a couple times a week, and here he was, ready to roll. I was stoked.

Jason is six years older than me. We never hung out as kids, because I was just his annoying little brother. Once I reached college, we built a better relationship. Jason leads by example and is a great older brother. He is a loving father and husband who truly enjoys his family. He also likes to have a good time.

After Limitless, my relationship with Jason improved even more. We are not only brothers but also good friends and hang out any chance we get.

Any time a runner would join us at this point of the run, I would chuckle; they didn't understand what we'd been through the past seventy-two hours.

"Is this the pace you're running?" Jason said, looking surprised.

Laughing, I said, "Dude, we are on mile two hundred. What do you expect?"

Two miles into Jason's run, I needed a short break, just enough time to eat a little and replenish our water bottles. After our short stop, my brother Josh decided to run with us. The three Levine brothers were running together. It hit me that we had never before run together.

"So what do you think of all this?" I asked Jason.

"I'm not sure yet. It's cool," Jason said, nonchalantly.

I laughed to myself. It took Jason about fifteen miles to fully understand the extremity and mission of this journey.

Hickey wanted my dad to run with us. He took the wheel of Jason's car so my dad could join us. My dad was an avid fitness enthusiast. He called me and shared his workouts with me. He'd say he had a great workout at California Fitness Academy, rode his bike ten miles, and swam a few laps. It made me happy that my dad was focused on being fit and healthy.

The Levine boys were running together for the first time in the Angeles National Forest. The four of us didn't spend much time together. Not that we did not want to, but with Jason living in the Bay Area and Josh living in Southern California, it was rare for all of us to be together just hanging out. Running that afternoon brought us together. That was a cool moment I would never forget.

We climbed the last hill of the Angeles National Forest, and, when we hit the top of the mountain, we stopped. From the Angeles National Forest lookout point, we could see Los Angeles below. It was one hell of a view! The elevation sign read 4,900 feet. That morning we had started at 2,700 feet. I had run thirty miles with 1,900 feet of elevation gain—a good spurt of running. To think that we had just run to the top of the Angeles National Forest from Visalia. Unbelievable! Looking down at LA renewed my outlook. Knowing we were getting closer to our final destination made me optimistic.

"Wow! We have run a long way," I said.

After a few minutes of enjoying the bird's-eye view and each other's company, we started the descent. I was usually light and fast running downhill, but my legs were so thrashed from running 230 miles, the downhill portion was punishing. After a fifteen-mile descent, the pavement eventually leveled off, which meant we were entering La Canada Flintridge, an actual city. I knew that when we reached this city, we had less than seventy miles left. It gave me hope.

The bustling city streets with cars whizzing by was a welcome sight, or so we thought. After running for three straight days with an accumulation of over 230 miles, taking on city streets wasn't the least bit enjoyable. The steep climbs of the Angeles National Forest were behind us, but we would soon be tested by unfore-seen obstacles of this journey.

Day 4 at 4:00 pm: 40 miles
Total: 234 miles

CHAPTER 16

....

LIFE THROWS CURVEBALLS

La Canada Flintridge to Sherman Oaks Starbucks

Jason was still running with us. His longest run to date was ten miles. He was close to reaching his initial goal of twenty-five miles. I was encouraged by watching him challenge his own self-limits. He was struggling. I could tell he was reaching his limit. But he kept pushing.

"I can run a little longer," Jason said repeatedly.

His was another inspiring story spurred on by this project.

Once we hit La Canada Flintridge, running became hectic. I wasn't sure of our exact route, but I figured we could just find our way through Los Angeles. This was poor planning on my part. It was about an eight-mile run from La Canada Flintridge to our next stop. Those eight miles were up and down for me. The city running didn't allow me to zone out because of having to navigate heavy traffic, wait at stoplights, and maneuver the city streets. To make matters worse, we lost our support team and the terrain was inconsistent. But with the help of Rocky directing our running route, we eventually made it to Glendale.

We had planned a dinner stop at Glendale Community College. It was a much-needed break, as I was hungry, and we had been running for countless hours. But on the journey, nothing really satisfied my hunger. Running sixteen hours a day and burning close to 13,000 calories, it had become difficult to keep pace with my famished state. Even as I ate, my hunger returned. I had to be careful not to overeat because it would affect my running. Stephanie did everything she could to vary the calories to keep me fueled. But sometimes she'd hand me food and I'd push it away because I didn't feel like what she was offering. Instead, I'd eat something small that sounded good, like a cookie, some peanut M&Ms, or a few gulps of Mountain Dew.

As I approached Glendale Community College, I hit a low point. I didn't know I was just two miles from the college, so I found some grass just off the side of the road and took a short break. After I downed a candy bar and sipped Gatorade, I lay down on the grass and closed my eyes for a few moments. The two-minute nap and food gave me a burst of energy. Rocky let me know we were a couple miles from the Community College. I couldn't get too comfortable at this stop. I laced my shoes and resumed running.

I was relieved to reach the college's parking lot. Both RVs were waiting for us with food, cold drinks, and chairs. I plunked down and, although tired, I was in good spirits. The crew was upbeat and ready for the rest of the journey. After a ten-hour day of running, I never knew what mood my team members would be in. I was happy to have positive people in my corner. Up to this point, there had never been any negative moments among the crew that I knew of. Everyone was dedicated to making the journey a positive experience.

Jason was right at twenty-seven miles. It was amazing to watch him chug along and tick away miles. He was resting, soaking his feet in ice water, and hoping to regain some energy to run a few more miles. As we were sitting and eating, I thought about the rest of the run. Actually, I had been thinking about this scenario the last few miles before reaching the college. It was close to 5:30

on Friday evening, and we were around mile 248. The initial goal was to be done at 10:00 a.m. I did the calculations in my head. We had fifty-two miles to go. I didn't want to go to sleep only to wake up with a sore body and have to run the next day.

So I devised a plan to keep running through the night. On the first day, we ran sixty-seven miles in about sixteen hours. That meant if we had around fifty-two miles to finish, we could come close to finishing by 10:00 a.m.

I called a meeting with the crew. They gathered around me as I soaked my feet in ice water and devoured a grilled ham-and-cheese sandwich, my favorite thing to eat on the journey. Something about the buttery bread and salty deli ham hit the spot.

I first thanked the crew for their selfless acts. It was humbling to know everyone was inspired and determined to assist with this project. I would not have been where I was without the team's help. I truly meant every word. Despite being sleep deprived and fatigued beyond measure, the endorphins and emotions were kicking in hard. For the first time, I had started to see the finish line. I was feeling unexpectedly ecstatic. So my excitement to create a plan to get there could not be contained. I felt like a football coach giving a half-time speech. I outlined the plan: to run through the night, only resting or sleeping when necessary. I needed everyone on board with positive attitudes. Any negativity would detract from the goal. Everyone appeared inspired and on board.

At this point, I'd like to highlight my incredible wife. I haven't sufficiently expressed my intense gratitude for her. Every man needs a rock by his side. Stephanie was that rock for me. She committed to this project without hesitation. She understood the commitment required to train and prepare for this event, and she supported me 100 percent. Stephanie wanted to help in any way she could. Leading up to the run, she helped with event fundraising and marketing. She tolerated my obsessive personality and my demanding training regimen. She understood when I had to sacrifice time away from the family.

During the journey, Stephanie was the behind-the-scenes hero. Because of her modesty, she wouldn't admit her critical importance to the overall success of the run. But she was an integral component to the journey. Five months pregnant, Stephanie drove the RV, took care of our JoJo, and fed me while running three hundred miles—not an easy feat! As the run was underway, she stayed busy preparing food. Food prep was a tough job, because food was a critical component of a successful journey. She also handled everything going on behind the scenes.

Once we decided to run through the night, Stephanie was completely supportive and by my side the entire time. I have said this before, but it bears repeating: Stephanie is by far my biggest support. I am so lucky to have such an understanding, loving, and caring wife.

Stephanie's journal excerpt on the plan to run through the night:

Pulling into the college parking lot with the RVs and seeing everyone hanging out was kind of a relief. Justin was resting and that was good because it had been a long day. I can only imagine how he is feeling. I'm getting pretty tired myself. Olivia is hanging in there with the help of Kim, Kelsey, and Suzin, Justin's mom. We all had some snacks, and Justin called a team meeting, so we all gathered around and calculated how much more he still had to go. It was about fifty miles! He said, "I say we just run through the night. How do you all feel about that?" I remember everyone looking around in silence, thinking, "Is he for real?" But I knew, just like he did, that this was what needed to be done. There was no question in my mind that he could do it, but it was more worrisome for me that he was going to run in the city. Everyone kept asking me if I was scared and worried that he was going to push too hard. Honestly, I have never seen so much determination in his eyes. "He will get it done. Don't worry," I said. I did not have time to worry unless he communicated to me that something might be wrong. Until then I would keep driving and making food.

Everyone was worried about me, because I was five months pregnant, taking care of Olivia, driving the RV, and making all of Justin's food. I told them I was fine and that I was going to be there until the end. No one was going to take that away from me. I'm sure I looked like crap 'cause I could feel it, but that didn't matter at that point. We were so close, yet so far away.

Before I knew it, I had eaten my sandwich, and it was time to pry myself from the chair and resume running. Getting out of the chair was becoming more and more difficult, as my legs would lock up after a few minutes of sitting. Like a disabled old man, I moaned as I made my way to my feet. I then changed into night-time running gear. Long sleeves, bright colors, new socks, and a headlamp, and I was ready to go. Changing clothes would be a fresh change of pace (no pun intended). It would feel like the start of a new run, and this helped my mindset.

As I walked around and got my legs moving, I asked for our secret weapon: chocolate-covered coffee beans. The previous three nights of sleeping had been restless, so I was extremely tired, but thanks to four or five coffee beans, I was pretty wound up. Despite the coffee-bean boost, my first few steps were challenging. I shuffled my feet like a ninety year old on a walker. The shuffle eventually morphed into a slow jog, and then into my normal ultra-running pace. Within a mile I was back into a rhythm. But this time was different. The anxiety of running through the night weighed heavily. My mind raced. *How would I respond?* The only time I had run through the night was the midnight to sunrise run, but I had not been running for three straight days leading up to that. *Would my body hold up?* How much worse could my body get? Hopefully no injuries would surface and stop me in my tracks. *How would*

I do without sleep? I had never gone this long with so little sleep. For the first few miles I was preoccupied by the unknowns of the upcoming night.

My thoughts were interrupted by heavy Los Angeles traffic. After two miles we lost our support vehicles and were dodging traffic and constantly stopping at traffic lights. It was frenzied running in fits and starts. It was impossible to hit my running zone and get lost in my thoughts. Having to weave in and out of traffic 250 miles into a run left me exasperated. Although delirium was setting in, we were actually aware of our safety. Hickey ran out in front, keeping an eye on cars. Jim was right by my side, talking as we ran.

Jason ran in front of me. His head was down and his feet were shuffling. He was obviously hitting his limit at nearly thirty miles. After about an hour of reckless running, we called Rocky and asked him to locate the vehicles. We had lost our cars and crew. I wasn't even sure we were headed in the right direction. In fact, we thought maybe we had just gone in circles. After around five or six miles of city running, we found a Starbuck's in Sherman Oaks, where we decided to stop and wait for Rocky. We stayed for about twenty-five minutes, enough time to pee and down some coffee. The break was nice, but we were wasting time and not getting closer to our goal.

When Rocky found us, we were tired and annoyed. We just wanted to run, but the traffic mayhem made it nearly impossible to route us correctly. I was definitely not the best person to be doing the navigation. Up to this point, we had followed my planned route almost to the T, but this city running was more than we bargained for.

Jason called it a night after having run thirty-one miles that day. His body was undoubtedly wrecked, but what an adventure.

My brother was relieved to be done. I was so proud of what he had accomplished.

Fueled by coffee and a snack, we slowly jogged away from Starbucks. I turned down the street where I thought Rocky had directed me to go. I ran about half a mile, looked over my shoulder, and saw Rocky in a full sprint chasing me down.

"Wrong way, Justin," he said, trying to catch his breath.

Oh, crap! Now I was really annoyed. We were wasting more time. We made a U-turn and headed back to Starbucks. On the walk back, I shifted into problem-solving mode.

"Let's figure this out, guys," I said to a frustrated Hickey and Rocky. I pulled up a map on my phone and identified an alternate route to get to our three-hundred mile mark. The plan I proposed to the crew was to pack up our cars and drive up to Camarillo, around fifty-five miles from Santa Monica. The downside was that the drive would take about sixty minutes. But once we were there, we could run right down Highway 1, a straight shot to our final destination. No more crazy traffic or trying to find our way on frenzied city streets. Talk about throwing a wrench in the plans. But the smooth, safer running would make it all worthwhile.

We took a vote and, with a majority for the plan, the decision was made to head to Camarillo. Hickey's wife was now with us at Starbucks. She carted a trunk full of goodies—cold fruit, Cliff bars, and beef jerky. These snacks were lifesavers. The rest of the crew was a few minutes away, parked at a nearby elementary school. We planned to meet them and then head to Camarillo.

We met up with the RVs and announced our change of plans. Lee, who was driving one of the RVs, had to get home. Lee had been invaluable, volunteering his time and allowing us to use his RV. At every rest and food stop, Lee would prop up chairs, get the drinks ready, and place a throw rug on the ground. Even though

I had just met Lee, he felt like part of my family for those three days.

We were now down to one RV and two vehicles.

The sun was down, darkness set in, and our adventure would now go into the depths of the night.

Day 4 at 8:00 p.m.: 59 miles

Total: 253 miles

CHAPTER 17

······························

A DEEP NIGHT OF RUNNING

We needed to gas up the RV, so the first stop was at a nearby gas station just before getting on the freeway to Camarillo. While we were refueling, my good buddy, Ira, just happened to pull up next to us. It was good to see a fresh face at this point in the run. It was especially good to see my friend Ira.

Ira and I had been close friends for over ten years. Ira was that guy you wanted on a Vegas trip because you knew he would make it memorable. We had partied hard together. We had gotten tattoos together. He was not only game for a good time; he was also genuine. I could talk to him about anything, and the authenticity of our relationship was what I liked most. We weren't afraid to tell each other the truth or what was on our minds. We respected each other and were there for each other in need. Ira was about to embark on his own Limitless journey.

During our drive to Camarillo, I ate, drank fluids, and rested my legs. I was too amped to take a nap or even to close my eyes. I was euphoric about the night ahead. I talked nonstop, rambling really. It was probably gibberish to everyone around me. Caffeine, food, and a short break helped me regain essential energy for the crazy-ass night ahead. I was trying to calculate our running mileage and identify our route while eating as much food as possible.

Before we knew it, we had arrived on the north side of Camarillo. We parked in a shopping center and prepped for our next leg.

It was 9:30 p.m. and we were at mile 253. Since we had wasted about an hour getting to Camarillo, the goal time for completion was pushed back to noon the next day. Honestly, at this point, the goal was to just finish. I stepped out of the RV to give Ira a big handshake and pat on the back. What we were about to withstand was unimaginable.

Hickey was spent. No one else was ready to run with me. When Ira was asked if he was ready to run, he hesitated at first. Ira's uncertainty quickly shifted into the cockiness that we all knew and loved.

"I don't give a shit. I'll do it," he said.

Ira was an athlete. He had done everything from motor biking, mountain biking, and mixed martial arts to a couple sprint triathlons and was now attempting an ultra-run. Ira wasn't an endurance athlete, though. He had probably run six miles a couple times before, so his running foundation was minimal. Even though he said he didn't care, I knew he really did care. This was his toughman reaction.

Ira changed into some borrowed running gear from Hickey. The only running shoes Ira had were his New Balance Minimus, shoes that gave a runner a barefoot feel but were durable enough for running. I didn't think they were meant for ultra-running. But they were the only shoes he had.

I was still amped from the caffeine I had been drinking during the drive, so my energy tank was full. Ira was also ready to go. We said a quick prayer in the parking lot, and ran into the night. The crew clapped their hands and wished us well as we took off. It seemed as if my adrenaline—energized delirium—had rubbed off on the group.

We started at our normal ultra-pace of five-and-a-half mph and my legs felt strong. We punched out those first sixty minutes easily. Our engaging conversation helped time pass quickly. We told Stephanie, who was still driving the RV, to meet us up the road just before merging onto Highway 1. We would take a short food break and get ready for the midnight run. We ran those first eight miles pretty strongly and before we knew it, we had arrived at the RV.

As we ate snacks and chatted, Ira said, "I'm running the rest with you. I don't give a shit."

I chuckled sarcastically. "Hold on. Just knock out a few more miles and then we'll see."

"No, I am going the rest of the way," he said.

Ira had never run farther than six miles. We were now eight miles into his run, and he had made up his mind to run another thirty-nine. This had happened all week. My support runners would come into the journey not knowing their future. They each had their limitations, but when they ran, a spiritual motivation emerged. When their bodies rebelled, their determination would kick in and keep them going. I was inspired anytime this would happen, and it would push me forward, closer to my goal. Knowing Ira would push himself to the brink in support of this journey was remarkable.

Our pit stop before embarking on Highway 1 was a blast. We wolfed down Top Ramen, hard-boiled eggs, a couple of chocolate chip cookies, and drank fluids. Ira was his jokester self, Jim danced, and I basked in the moment. Hickey forced me to consume more food so I would stay fueled up. I was stoked for this next epic section of running and Ira was determined to run fifty-six miles. Determination, purpose, and motivation soared. Around midnight, we took off on Highway 1.

We merged onto the highway, moved over to the shoulder, and began our wild Pacific Coast Highway (PCH) run. Running into the depths of the night was spooky. If it were not for our head-lamps beaming down on the road, we could barely see a few steps ahead of us. I remember listening to Ira's stories. He talked like he had just taken a toke, but in my delirious state, it actually made sense. To most, it would have sounded like crazy talk.

"Life is crazy, bro. To be out here in the middle of the night, running. This is crazy, yet exhilarating. Most people don't get it. They live their lives just to get by, missing so many opportuni-ties. Here, we're pushing ourselves to a deeper level," Ira said. I intently listened as we ran.

A dark, misty, and long highway led us to our destination. It was an unforgettable moment. It is said that ultra-running is ninety percent mental, and the last ten percent is in your head. I started to feel physical pain thirty miles into the run and, if I wanted to keep going, I would have to somehow distance myself from the pain. I had to mentally talk myself into pushing beyond physical suffering. How much mental anguish could I handle? My body had hit its limits back in Tehachapi, but my mind and my spirit transported me. Physical pain was guaranteed to sur-face. But could I mentally erase the pain and shift into a state of bliss? The vicious cycle of euphoria and depression became the norm. I couldn't enjoy my runner's high for long; a state of despair would quickly negate any elation. Running long distances was like therapy. You were inside your head. You reflected on life. And weaknesses surfaced. Depression set in. But when you pushed through, your mind strengthened, your spirit rose, and happiness entered. And you lived to see another day. For me, running was a perfect analogy of how I should live.

As we continued to run into the depths of the night, I became disoriented, lost in a dream-like state. At times, I completely lost my perception of reality. Ira and I bumped shoulders due to sleep deprivation and periodically talked nonsense. When I asked for water, Ira handed me a water bottle. All the while, Jim silently rode his bike. From 12:30 a.m. to 2:00 a.m. Jim didn't say a word, which was unusual for him. He battled his own fatigue and exhaustion. Riding a bike at five-and-a-half miles per hour for three hundred miles wasn't easy. But Jim was a warrior. He entered the battle with us as a soldier and would do anything for his team. He stayed by my side every step of the way. Jim was one of the most selfless human beings I knew, and I tried my best to emulate him.

Between 2:00 a.m. and 3:30 a.m. we ran in a trance state. Step-by-step we progressed, suspending our minds away from our bodies. Ultra-runners refer to out-of-body experiences. I was having a strong episode, slipping in and out of my own physical presence. It was as if my mind floated above, peering down at my body, and physically I was no longer in control. My mind would somehow guide my body to move forward.

We trotted without exchanging a word. Eerie skies loomed overhead. Ocean waves crashed as if talking to us. My eyes were heavy and my body was fatigued. My mind would go in and out of being in the zone and being tempted to stop. Not quit, but stop and rest. Rollercoaster emotions yo-yoed through my body in minutes. I shared my mental battles with Ira.

"Just keep running. Think of it like this: you are just out on the coastal highway running," he said. It helped me move another step forward. I took one step at a time, not knowing where my mental state would carry me.

It was approaching 3:30 a.m. and we decided to take a pit stop. This was the most intense aid station of the entire trip. We were all depleted of energy and strength, not just from running but also from the lack of sleep. When we arrived at the RV, I snuggled down on the dirt canvas. I didn't care anymore. I elevated my feet on a chair to reduce the swelling. Within seconds a cup of soup was in my hand. And then a chocolate chip cookie. Don't ask me who handed me the food. All I knew was that I taking in much-needed calories. Food became very unemotional for me, almost mechanical. I no longer ate for taste. I ate for necessity—anything that would propel me one more step. I would repeatedly say, "I'm starving." We'd break, I'd eat four hundred to eight hundred calories, run a few miles, and then I'd be famished again. The problem was I was burning more than I could take in. Hunger was a constant the last one hundred miles.

While I rested my eyes, Rocky worked on my feet. It was lightly raining, so Kent Moore, my PR manager, held an umbrella over me. He had been busy back home updating my Facebook page. We sent him text messages, and he would relay those messages through Facebook to keep supporters in the loop. Kent wanted to see the final hours up close and personal, so he joined us.

Kent shared his thoughts in a journal entry:

I found them on Highway 1 at 2:00 a.m. Justin has a road crew that is a well-oiled machine. Imagine a NASCAR pit crew just for Justin. I came in right as he was taking a quick break to get food and put on clean clothes. At 3:30 a.m. it had started to rain, just enough to get everything wet. I could tell Justin was beyond tired. But I could also see from the determination in his face that he wasn't going to stop, and if you asked him to, he would probably just smile and keep running. It was one thing to get texts or phone calls, but to actually see this event happening, well let's just say, I believe in Limitless.

Rocky worked my feet, Stephanie cooked me pancakes, Kimmie fed me those pancakes, and the rest of the crew huddled around us, tiredly, watching my doldrums.

My sister had joined us.

As we approached the stop I said, "Liz, good to see you." She smiled, but I could see the concern in her eyes. "Pretty crazy, huh?"

"Uh, yeah," she said, sarcastically.

At this point, I looked pretty weathered. The few wrinkles under my eyes were pronounced due to sleep deprivation, and my hair was greasy, messed up, and knotted. My sister told me later I looked worn and tattered and at least ten years older.

As the rain fell, I closed my eyes for a few more minutes. It seemed like just seconds. It felt so good to rest my eyes, but, the minute it started to feel good, I snapped out of it, opened my eyes, sat up and said, "Okay, it's time to go again." At 3:30 a.m. I struggled to put into words my feelings. I felt inebriated yet I was completely sober and aware of my surroundings. This definitely is turning into a great movie," I told Josh. At least my sense of humor was still intact.

I pushed myself up and headed into the RV to use the restroom. One of the best indications of dehydration is urine color. If my urine had been dark yellow—close to brown—then I would have needed to quickly replenish my fluids. My urine was a light lemonade color. I was relieved to see my pee was normal. I was doing a good job of drinking fluids to maintain normal hydration levels. Water alone wasn't sufficient, though. Maintaining proper electrolyte balance was critical for hydration. When sodium levels became dangerously low, hyponatremia could occur. Drinking too much water in endurance sports could dilute my sodium, and my body's water levels could elevate, which would swell my cells. Mild to life-threatening health conditions could occur. This was a component that as an endurance athlete I needed to pay attention to. I made sure to drink fluids and consume electrolytes to prevent problems from developing. We kept an eye on my urine color to catch problems early.

While in the bathroom, I looked in the mirror and said out loud, "Holy shit, I look bad." I chuckled to myself. What did I expect? I had put myself through the ringer. I glared into my sleep-deprived eyes. I needed to dig deep within my soul for this last stretch of running. I splashed cold water on my face and threw some water on my hair to clean it up. I made my way back outside. It was time to go again. What seemed like a thirty-minute break was only about ten minutes. Tired was a gross understatement. Sore underestimated how my body felt. But thankfully I still had the keep-going mentality. I wasn't sure how to specifically train for this state of mind. To put my body through this degree of anguish and do it numerous times for training was a bit absurd. I was a newbie in the ultra-distance world and unfamiliar with these deep emotions.

After getting some much-needed rest and recovery, Hickey rejoined the group. At this point his ultra-running experience was needed. He recounted a story about his one-hundred-mile Pine to Palm ultra-race. He said he ran through the night, fighting his body not to stop. As tiredness crept in, he leaned on a big tree, closed his eyes for two minutes, and then suddenly woke up and resumed running. He did this several times during the night until the sun rose, which generated essential energy. I couldn't wait for daylight. This had been the longest night of my life and sunrise was still a few hours away.

We returned to Highway 1 and I immediately went back into a running trance. Our conversations were abbreviated. In fact, we did not talk much during this section. The rhythmic waves lulled us into a hypnotic state. We did our best to zone out and put one foot in front of the other. Nearing twenty-five miles, Ira was uncharacteristically quiet. I knew he was hurting and his mind was experiencing the effects of long-distance running. Jim was quiet too. Hickey was in good spirits, but he always seemed to find a smile in the toughest of times.

Nine months before Limitless, Hickey was out on a regular training bike ride. He was preparing for a big race season ahead. In addition to Limitless, he had plans to race in a few half-Ironmans and ultra-running races that year. During the leg of the ride, his breathing was labored. He was puzzled as to why it had become so erratic. He stopped on the side of the road, took a few deep breaths, rested, and tried to continue. But he couldn't. Later that day he went to the doctor. The doctor told Hickey he had exercise-induced asthma, gave him medication, and sent him on his way. But his condition worsened overnight. He wheezed and had difficulty breathing while trying to sleep, so his wife took him to the ER. Within twelve hours, he was in surgery for a pneumothorax, or a punctured lung.

I visited him after his surgery. It was the first time I had seen a down and dejected Hickey, but amazingly he still had a smile on his face. On the table next to his hospital bed were running and triathlon magazines, smoothies, and hospital equipment. He was planning his next epic adventure from the hospital.

"I'm going to run the Rim to Rim to Rim in the Grand Canyon in a few months."

"Just get healthy, brother, and take small steps to recovery," I said.

Hickey was filled to the brim with enthusiasm. His enthusiasm was contagious; he was the kind of person you wanted on your side. Two months after the doctor cleared him to exercise he was running the Grand Canyon.

Hickey expresses thoughts that reveal his nature:

We limit our own self-development if we are distracted by society's perceived deficiency. I may not be the fastest, but God has blessed me with endurance and putting your talent to work builds enduring character. No doubt, in a society driven by luxury and modern-day conveniences, choosing the discomfort of running, let alone ultra-running is "weird." But now is the time in my life when I can do this. My health is my wealth. When my doctor cleared me to run after my pneumothorax surgery, I became a runner again, and through my actions, I joined the Limitless journey to inspire others to dream more, learn more, do more, and become more. Running has its highs and its lows, and you do the best you can, where you are, with what you have now. You work at it with all your heart and reach past your limits with a positive attitude.

The dark coastal sky mesmerized me, but deep fatigue had set in. It was around 4:30 a.m., and I was crashing. We had been running for forty-five minutes since our last stop.

I noticed a bush on the side of the road, and I said, "Man, I am tired. I just need five minutes snuggled up to that bush, and I'll be okay."

"I think it would be a good idea for us to lie down for a few minutes to rest our eyes. We can rest for forty-five minutes, regain some energy, and then we can start running when the sun rises. That will spark our energy," said Hickey.

I wasn't arguing at this point. I desperately needed a short nap. Even lying down in a bed for twenty minutes would have done wonders.

We would run another ten minutes to the RVs parked on the side of the highway. We had decided everyone would nap for an hour. This would hopefully rejuvenate our crew. We ran up to the RV.

Hickey announced, "We're going to rest and sleep for an hour, no more. Everyone needs to take it easy and close their eyes. Then we'll continue on."

I didn't say a word. I hurried to the back of the RV, slipped off my shoes, and nestled into bed. Trying to get to sleep was nearly impossible. Achy joints, burning and inflamed muscles, and a fried immune system made falling asleep tough. I closed my eyes for fifteen minutes. I tossed and turned for another five minutes, and I just lay there, eyes wide open, for another ten minutes. Then my mind took over. *I need to go run. Man, I am tired. Only a marathon to go. Shit, a marathon to go.* The heaviness of depression was taking hold. But I then sat up. I shivered. It felt like the flu was coming on. Somehow I managed to pry myself out of bed. I stood up and headed to the bathroom. I looked fiercely at my drowsy eyes in the mirror. "Son of a bitch, finish this," I said aloud. I slapped my cheeks and threw some cold water on my face, drenched my hair, dried off and left the bathroom.

When I entered the narrow corridors of the RV, I experienced another sudden onset of depression. I gazed around the RV. Everyone was resting or slowly moving because they heard me stirring. I witnessed everyone's fatigue, stress, and deprivation. They were sacrificing for me, for this project. Damn, I felt bad. I toasted an English muffin, spread peanut butter and jelly on it, poured myself a small cup of coffee, and sat and ate in silence. Somehow I managed to step outside the RV.

My body was on overdrive and my feet were throbbing, but I knew I needed to tick off the miles. Quitting wasn't an option and never even entered my mind. I could have stopped right there. I had just run 275 miles. Truly commendable. But quitting was the easy road. I had never taken that road in my life. I fought for my goals and the things that were important to me. Sometimes my stubbornness caused conflict. That was okay because my passion to live was what fueled my life. I admit I had to have obsessive tenacity to achieve this goal. Nothing was going to get in my way. Mental lows, physical pain, or a sleep-deprived body—none of that would stop me from this mission. I continued to find a way to push myself out of mental roadblocks to enable me to continue.

A goal awaited me and my determination kept me moving forward. At 5:30 a.m. the ocean air was so chilly, I slipped on a vest and arm warmers. As I waited for the others, I stood on the side of the road and battled my thoughts. *Go, Justin. Rest, Justin. Go. Rest. Go.* All I needed to do was to start running, but I just stood there, paralyzed. I stared at the dark skies, bemused by my current state. The sky reflected my physical and mental state. Josh approached me and threw his arm around me. He could see the extreme fatigue and emotional toll this run had taken on me.

With a weary voice I said, "I am at my brink, man. I am at my brink." I continued gazing out at the road, my eyes filled with tears. I crossed my arms and shivered when I noticed that Josh was crying. I couldn't understand what he was saying. But I knew he, too, was determined to complete this project. We were all emotionally shattered. This pivotal moment was one I would never forget. It was then that I fully grasped the amplitude of this journey.

Although worn, tattered, and mentally spent, emotion hit me like a bolt of lightning, and I took off running. I was crying but setting my fastest pace yet.

As I took off, Josh yelled, "Get it done, brother!" I harnessed my emotion to strengthen and propel me. Sometimes in life, you must run as fast as you can. No matter the pain, the anguish I might have felt, or the curveballs this journey had thrown at me, my best solution was to run fast. I needed to dig deep and, in doing so, I found myself once again.

I was running fast, the fastest of the entire journey. I couldn't stand on the side of the road anymore. I needed to go, and that is what I did. Those first few minutes felt effortless. As I was light on my feet and my leg turnover was high, I beamed. I actually chuckled. *This is crazy shit.* In minutes I went from depression to exhilaration. It was surreal. I ran alone for about a mile, and then I glanced back and saw Hickey trying to catch up. I slowed and he caught up with me. Then Jim joined us. The three amigos were together again.

"Don't worry, guys. I'm good to go," I said.

Five miles later I needed to use the restroom, so we stopped at a convenience store. I bought a soda and guzzled it down. I desperately needed the sugar. When I exited the store, I noticed that Kimmie and Ira had rejoined us. They told me that they had been running hard trying to catch us.

At 6:30 a.m., we were anxious for daylight. Sunrise meant we would be closer to our final destination. We all anticipated the final morning of running to the Santa Monica Pier. But we still had about twenty miles to go. We had just completed ten-and-a-half marathons over the past four days. Twenty miles seemed attainable, but I remained humble and focused on the goal.

I was stoked to have a small running group of Hickey, Ira, Kimmie, and Kelsey. The group's energy was contagious. I needed all the support and positivity to tackle these final miles. My running group carried my water. They asked if I needed anything. They walked when I walked. Knowing others were pushing their own individual limits motivated and inspired me. I probably didn't tell my pace-team enough, but I was truly appreciative of their friendship and support throughout Limitless. These runners sacrificed time away from their families and endured physical and mental anguish for this mission. I was honored to have them by my side.

Day 5 at 6:30 am
Total: 280 miles

CHAPTER 18

....

DETERMINATION IS STRONGER THAN WEAKNESS

We headed into Malibu as daylight approached. Unfortunately, the coastal clouds lingered throughout the morning and obscured the sun. I had been looking forward to sunlight, but any daylight was better than darkness. We had completed a good chunk of running since our early-morning nap. Miles were ticking away. Rolling hills along the Pacific Coast Highway made for tough but fun running. I would walk or jog most of the hills and let momentum propel me down the hill. Around 7:30 a.m. we took a break. We plopped down on the side of Highway 1, eating food and enjoying the good feeling as cars zoomed by. The drivers were probably thinking: what the heck are these guys doing? If they only knew. This pit stop was a positive one. Endorphins were soaring and we were all feeling on top of the world. I appreciated my running high and relished the moment. Hickey and Ira iced their feet, experiencing the effects of ultra-running.

"What is this? Justin should be the one icing," Rocky said. Running through the night had been torturous. We hadn't had many high moments in the past several hours, so we basked in this one fleeting bright spot.

Running now was about moving forward. My pace slowed as my feet shuffled along. It was more of a hobble than a run. As we approached Malibu, I had my first realization that our journey was nearing the end. Earlier in the morning, there had been rumors of a group of friends waiting for us in Malibu. When I glanced down the road, I saw a group of people just off the highway waiting for us. I was stoked to see everyone. When we reached the large group of supporters, although I didn't show it, I was thrilled to run with everyone. I had a focused, deadpan expression, because I knew we still had thirteen miles to run and I was completely spent. Next thing I knew, we had ten people running with us down Highway 1. Friends from Visalia, a couple buddies from San Diego, and random runners from Facebook joined in for the last thirteen miles. It was a great scene.

Ira ran with his head down right next to me. He had never run six miles before, and he was now on mile thirty-four! He was battling his own physical and mental barriers. But, just like me, he kept moving forward. The human spirit was pretty amazing and the power I witnessed throughout the journey was incredible.

Hickey's spirits were high. He lived for this atmosphere. He was in the middle of the group, telling tales of our adventure, and laughing. Although my excitement didn't show, deep down I needed this group of runners. I was battling so hard inside, and I needed them to piggyback me through the final half marathon.

The next three to five miles were rough. My emotional roller-coaster intensified. I walked when I snacked. Literally it seemed that one mile I would feel strong and positive, and the very next I hit a wall and felt dejected and down. My mind combatted mental anguish and physical duress. I was pretty beaten up, but, with the support of my crew, I kept putting one foot in front of the other.

We ran in a tightly-knit formation. I listened to the excited chatter behind me. Trying my best to keep my emotional rollercoaster to myself, I managed a few conversations with fellow runners. I bonked pretty hard with only about ten miles to go. We took a break in the parking lot of Duke's restaurant in Malibu. I just needed to sit down and take in some food. I downed an Odwalla bar and two small tangerines. Aching and sore from the day before, Jason asked me how I was doing. I repeated the same question to him.

"It's like a truck hit me," said Jason. I chuckled. Jason had his iPad, and his two sons were on Skype wanting to say hi to me. My nephews gave me a jolt of energy. When my low points would strike, I needed just a few minutes to regain my composure. If it was strictly a food thing, the solution was to consume calories, which would increase my blood sugar levels, and I'd be recharged. But mostly it was a mind thing, and I needed a few minutes of solitude to alleviate the depression. It was so much like real life.

After my snack and short break, I felt a small burst of energy. I got back up and continued running. We ran two miles and reached another parking lot, where I stopped for a few minutes, drank some Gatorade, and ate a Nutrigrain bar. At this stop, runners, supporters, and my crew members encircled me. It must have been more than twenty people. People analyzed my every move. I wore my sunglasses to cover up my droopy, bloodshot eyes. I was usually a confident person, but at this moment, I was overcome with insecurity.

Running the next mile was excruciating. With six miles to go, I slammed into a wall like nothing I had ever felt before. It was the toughest wall of my three-hundred mile run. Sleep deprived. Weak. Mentally crushed. Vulnerable. I hung on by a thin thread. I had less than a 10k to run, but would I be able to do it?

The group dispersed as I headed into the RV. I needed to be alone and sit quietly. At first, Stephanie, my dad, and sister just stared at me, waiting for me to talk. I said nothing. Instead, I sat motionless and groaned.

"Are you okay?" asked Stephanie. Her brow was knitted with worry.

"Yeah, just give it time," I said.

"Are you sure?" said my dad.

"Yeah. These walls have been happening on and off the past thirty miles. It will run its course, and I'll be fine," I said.

Stephanie handed me some apple slices. I was so fatigued, I could barely eat them. But I knew I needed the calories, so I forced them down. Hickey brought me a cup of coffee to keep caffeine in my bloodstream. Anything would help at this point. Ira appeared and took a seat right next to me, probably feeling the exact same way. We both stared into a daze as if lost. I suppose we were a bit lost, lost in the moment of this extreme expedition. We had descended into an abyss, and honestly, I didn't know if we had the strength to climb out.

Determination was a strong character trait. Many people gave in to weakness because it was more comfortable than enduring hardship. Determination pushed me out of my comfort zone.

Although it would have been tempting to give in, I had a goal to achieve, and my willpower kept me going, no matter how uncomfortable I became. In that moment, I eliminated quitting from my mind. Not finishing was not an option. Attaining my goal, no matter the struggle or fight that I was going through, was my only choice.

With much anguish, I straightened my posture and stood up, took a deep breath, and left the RV. I knew I just needed to get moving. First I started walking. Walking turned into a slow jog, and a slow jog turned into my ultra-running pace. "There he goes," someone said when the other runners realized I had taken off. Hurriedly they caught up with me. We ran in a cluster into Santa

Monica. I was doing everything to sustain my energy and keep moving—a gel, a shot block, sips of soda. *One step at a time.* I was pretty subdued and quiet while I focused my energy on running. It was then I noticed a hot spot—a possible blister—on my left foot. I was 295 miles in and my first blister was surfacing. I summoned the blister squad: Rocky. We laughed at the fact that my first blister had appeared so late into the run. He did his magic, taped up the blister, and I was good to go.

When I began running, I looked out into the distance, and I spotted the famous Santa Monica pier and the Ferris wheel on the horizon. This was a welcome sight and motivated me to pick up the pace. We were approaching three hundred miles. But we weren't there yet. Some local runners joined us and suggested we take the bike and run route that followed the coastline. I liked this plan, as it would make for a safer run than running on a busy highway. We made our way down to the coastal path, where we passed other runners and cyclists. For most of them, it was just a normal run on the beach. For us, it was the last few miles of a wild adventure. As we ran by the weekend warriors, I said, "They have no clue where our run started."

We were now three miles to the finish. The plan was to meet up with two police officers on motorcycles, and they would escort us to the pier. I wasn't fit to be making executive decisions regarding the route.

I said to Josh, "Just have them get us there in the shortest and easiest route possible." Josh was probably not the right person to be making these decisions either. I wasn't sure who was more spent: him or me.

Ignoring my request for an easy route, the police officers led us up steep hills and around corners. It seemed as if they were doing the exact opposite of my initial request. But these miles got us closer to our three-hundred-mile mark. I remained positive because I knew the end was near.

Ira fell off the group's pace. He hobbled, struggling to finish with us, but the energy of the group picked him up and kept him going. The last couple miles were bittersweet. As much as I wanted to be done, I also wanted to cherish these last few moments as much as I could. Positivity was in the air and everyone was happy.

We climbed our last hill, a pretty tough incline, turned the corner and ran parallel with the beach. We arrived at Ocean Avenue in Santa Monica, a running hotspot. It was the finish of the famous Los Angeles Marathon. On Saturdays and Sundays hundreds of locals ran there. A few local runners spontaneously joined our group. Friends filled them in, "This guy, Justin, just ran from Visalia." We had about twenty people running the final stretch with us, which made for an unforgettable finish.

We finally arrived at a section of the Santa Monica park. In my best Forrest Gump impression, I said, "This is good. I'm done." I stopped right there and the run was over.

Visalia to Santa Monica: 102 hours

Total: 300 miles

CHAPTER 19

....

EMOTIONS

had always been able to hide my emotions, but after I finished, I was overcome with emotion. I first wanted to hug and kiss Stephanie and JoJo. Once I found them, I gave them a huge embrace. Of course JoJo didn't know what was going on, so she pushed me away. I was delighted to hug and kiss my wife. I could not have achieved this goal without her.

Jim approached me and we both cried as we embraced. Jim never left my side. And he never stopped smiling. His support was remarkable. Knowing how much he sacrificed for this adventure was truly humbling. I was thrilled to have him on my team.

Next, I spotted Rocky. He was such an integral part of this run. Not only did he keep my body functioning, but his enduring support was essential. He remained positive and was willing to help the team in any way he could.

Hickey soaked in the positive energy of the group as everyone clustered in the park. Hickey fought through fatigue, long nights, and physical pain to be my number-one pace runner. He ended up running 210 miles with me. Who did that? Josh Hickey did. We have a life-long friendship. We continue to train, talk fitness, and enjoy beers together. He will always have a special place in my heart for his courage during Limitless.

Ira was relishing the moment as well. I couldn't believe what he had just done. His body was in pain, but he showed courage and grit in stepping up to help a friend. I will never forget Ira's amazing Limitless journey. I exchanged hugs and high-fives with everyone. We laughed and cried and beamed; sometimes all three simultaneously. It was surreal to have reached the finish line. Someone handed me an ice-cold chocolate milk and I chugged it as fast as I could.

We posed for a few group pictures. I personally thanked everyone who ran the last section with us. What a moment it was! My body was numb, but quickly the deep soreness permeated. I hobbled to take a seat on the grass. We huddled together, enjoying each other, the sand, and the sea. The ocean waves crashed in the background and the positive vibes abounded. It was one of those times that you wish would never end. I would have relished it longer if I hadn't been starving, exhausted, and ready for a shower. It took every last ounce of strength for me to stand up. I gingerly walked to the RV, where a steaming pizza was waiting for me. I crushed as many slices as I could get down—probably in record time. My good friend Brian Hyde (the tall guy who talked to me at the beginning of the run) called me, and the minute we started talking, tears streamed down my cheeks. Emotion set in pretty quickly.

All I could think about was a warm shower. After an hour of hanging out at the park, I went to Josh's house, two miles from the beach. I've never enjoyed a shower as much. In fact, I sat down and let the water stream down my body. My legs were so sore and my feet were completely swollen, I didn't want to stand. After the shower, I ate more and lay down for a much-deserved nap.

CHAPTER 20

....

RECOVERY AND BEYOND

The night after I finished the run, we stayed in a hotel room for the night. I iced my swollen feet once an hour for ten minutes throughout the night. My aching, pulsating feet and legs made falling asleep difficult. All night, I felt blood rushing to my feet. I woke up in the morning extremely sore and tired. I was ready to go home. But before we left, I took another long, hot shower. As the warm water soothed my body, waves of elation washed over me. I did it! Three hundred miles! I was filled with relief that it was over.

We packed our bags and headed home. Stephanie drove, Jim took shotgun, and I sat in the back with my legs propped up on blankets and pillows—in full-on recovery mode. We made a pit stop at McDonalds to quell my hunger. On the menu that day was a cheeseburger, a twenty-piece chicken nugget meal, large fries, and a chocolate shake. You could say I indulged a bit.

The week after I finished I iced my legs and feet, ate outlandish amounts of food, and gave into plain ol' laziness. I didn't even think about running, working out, or doing anything active. I just wanted to lie around the house and reminisce about the journey. I was caught off guard by the waves of positive emotions that hit me. When reflecting on the journey, I'd be overcome with tears. These positive emotions continued to hit me for weeks after the run and still give me goosebumps when I think of my incredible adventure.

Two weeks after finishing Limitless, I put JoJo in the running stroller, and we ran eight miles to the local farmer's market. This normally easy run felt like twenty miles. I knew then that I was not ready to run yet, so I allowed another two weeks to go by before I resumed running. I instead incorporated weightlifting, light cycling, and stretching sessions into my routine. This allowed me to move without pounding my body. I took a week off work. After a week, I was happy to return to work and my normal routine.

Six weeks after we finished the run, we held a charity event to hand over a check to the Central Valley Team in Training group. Limitless raised $16,000 for the Leukemia and Lymphoma Foundation. Handing over a check for this amount was exhilarating. It was remarkable what a group of positive people were capable of doing when we put our minds together and worked for a common cause.

Limitless was created to generate positivity and the I-can-do-anything mindset. The mission was achieved and it is only the beginning of sharing this message. This three-hundred-mile run was physically demanding and the hardest thing I have ever done, but the effects it had on my mental and spiritual being changed the way I viewed life. I was deep in the trenches of running, battling through tough mental spots, confronting my weaknesses, and fighting physical anguish, but as I chiseled my way through each low spot, life became increasingly better. I truly believe that anything is possible and I ran three hundred miles to prove this philosophy. Did I come back a changed person? Absolutely! The whole experience was humbling, as I was able to witness people come together for a common goal. People who ran with me broke their own barriers. It demonstrated how powerful the human spirit is, especially when positive people come together. I came back with a better appreciation of the people in my life and the relationships I have built.

Did doubt ever enter my mind? Absolutely. My mind played tricks on me at times, especially deep into the run when I was sleep deprived, hungry, and my body ached. But quitting never crossed my mind. People told me that they still saw burning determination in my eyes at mile 250. Failure was not an option. I was going to finish. I just needed to allow the low spots to play out, because every low spot was followed by a high spot, which kept me going forward.

My deep passion continues to challenge others to build a personal belief system and inspires people to live life to the fullest. I have high aspirations to help people stretch their limits and to reach their own ultimate way of life. I live for others and want to see people succeed. I like to see happiness on peoples' faces. I want people to achieve their goals. I want others to believe that anything is possible! This is my mission and I will spread this message for the rest of my life.

The Limitless life is possible. Let's go for it one step at a time.

FACEBOOK MOTIVATION

....

I was so humbled and inspired by the support and encouragement I received on my Facebook page that I wanted to share some of the messages.

You are absolutely amazing! I have been questioning myself for four days, how the human body can endure such a feat. I'm not sure how you do it but am so glad/proud that you are. I have had no motivation to work out or do a thing to better myself in years. You have made me think twice, three, and four times. If you can do what you've just done, I can do what I've always wanted to. Justin, I am beyond proud of you and so is Dad. I am now ready to turn my life around. And for that, I thank you. Good luck on the rest of your journey. –Lacey S.

OMG! You're almost there, Justin. We all knew you would do it. Good lesson in life. If you're facing some difficulties, push ahead and things will get better. Thank you for proving that to a lot of people these last five days. Love you. –Kathy, aka "Grandma"

I started running 5k runs last month and hope to do a half marathon next year. Today while running, all I saw in front of me was the word "Limitless." Thanks for the inspiration! –Chelsea S.

You've done a lot more on your journey than raise money for leukemia research. You've shown thousands, if not tens of thousands, of people that anything is possible if you put your blood, sweat, and time into something. You're a true inspiration to many. –Chad A.

Congratulations on the accomplishment of the journey you completed. I have no doubt your life is forever changed as a result of this journey. But I need to thank you for showing me that Limitless is available to us all, including me. Your journey has shown me beyond any doubt that Limitless living and goals are truly within my grasp. I look forward to seeing and chatting with you upon your return home. You are truly an amazing man, and the Lord blessed me by placing you in my life! –Lee

Arrived at the Limitless crew in Camarillo. Decided to run fifty-six miles with Justin in fifteen hours. We've been up for over twenty-four hours! This was an epic, life-changing journey with my brother from another mother. I cannot explain the emotional rollercoaster we went through. This experience has pushed me to a point I never thought I could achieve. Thank you to the support team. They are a beautiful group of people. Love you all. –Ira

Amazing and inspirational aren't words that cut the mustard anymore. You've moved "miles" beyond that, and I don't think there are words. Love you much—all of you! So proud of the whole team, spearheaded by you and your dream! –Debbie

You are an inspirational and amazing human being. If only more people were like you, this world would be a better place. –Renee

I say this with a smile on my face, and I'm sure I speak for all of us. You have touched our hearts in many ways, and we could not be any prouder of you. I have to say I have much respect and admiration for you.

Welcome home, Justin. Enjoy your time and relax with your beautiful wife and family. —Gabby

Congratulations Justin! I woke up at 5:30 this morning and went out for a seven-mile run with Limitless stuck in my head. Thanks to you, man. —Pedro

Shout out to Justin who is almost finished with his Limitless journey! Running three hundred miles from Visalia to the Santa Monica Pier in just four-and-a-half short days! You inspire me every day to believe in my-self and to live life without limits and I am so proud and blessed to have been trained by such an amazing person! Keep going Justin! Your story, will, determination, and attitude inspire people everywhere, every day. You are beyond amazing. You are Limitless! —Kayla

My good friend, Justin Levine, is working on completing his goal of running three hundred miles, from Visalia to Santa Monica. He is defi-nitely showing us what Limitless means! We are so proud of him! Please keep him in your prayers as he completes this awesome feat tonight and tomorrow! We love you, Justin. Wish we could be there to cheer you on, but will be in spirit! —Melissa

I can't really express the feelings I have. Maybe "inspired" is the best word to use. But there is a guy named Justin Levine and he is running three hundred miles, from Visalia to Santa Monica. It's really inspiring and has me captivated. It's a truly amazing feat. —Zann

When most people are walking away from their dreams, you're living yours! Simply amazing! —Julie

You are inspiring people you have never met. Your words and actions motivate others to make changes by pushing beyond the comfort zone. Beast mode. —Eric

ACKNOWLEDGEMENTS

....

MY HEROES

My wife, Stephanie, for always supporting and believing in me.

My three daughters, Olivia JoJo, Bobbi Jo, and our angel in heaven, Inspire.

My parents for instilling faith, determination, and a solid work ethic when I was a child. My mom drove a car, supporting this endeavor every step of the way. My dad even ran a few miles with me.

My brother Josh, for believing in this project and for being my best friend. Also for running with me the entire journey.

Josh Hickey, my number-one pace runner who ran 210 miles with me.

Jim Barnes, who rode his bike next to me, smiling and comforting me, all three hundred miles.

Rocky Ciseneros, my good friend, who took care of my body and kept me strong.

Shawn Taylor, who has done nothing but live life to the fullest, battled hip surgery and then ran twenty-six miles with me.

Eric Galvan, who trained, committed, and ran the first six miles with me.

Salina Marroquin, who ran the first nineteen miles with me.

Steve Juarez, the best man in my wedding and a great friend, who ran miles six to eighteen with me.

James Wilson, who ran the first twenty-four miles with me.

Eric Blain, my good friend, who met us in Porterville and ran thirty-one miles with me.

Tyler Baxley, who met up with us on the morning of Day 2 and ran into and through Bakersfield with me.

Landon Brokaw, who ran thirty miles with me. It was by far his longest run!

Lindsey Clemens, who was by my side for thirty-one miles, never faltering and staying positive.

Raul Gonzalez, who drove up from Visalia and ran with me in the Angeles National Forest.

Antonio Luevano, who drove up from Visalia. He kept me company as I battled some tough running lows.

Kelsey Schulte, who ran thirteen miles with me during the last three days. She also helped the crew get groceries, ice, and other items we needed for the run.

Kimmie Artiaga, my sister-in-law, who ran many spurts with me during the last three days.

My brother Jason, who drove down from his hometown to run with me on Day 4.

Ira Zermeno, who showed up at 9:00 p.m. on Friday and ran the last fifty-six miles with me.

Jamie Hickey, who helped with food, drinks, and car support the final three days.

My sister Elizabeth, who showed up at 2:00 a.m. on Saturday to be there for support. She even ran a couple miles to keep me company.

Lee Feickert, for driving and letting us use his RV and for his tremendous support.

Robin Twitty, for supporting and cheering us on during the last three days.

Kent Moore, my PR manager, who updated my Facebook page.

Dave Edwards, who was in the trenches getting footage for the documentary.

Aunt Josie for taking the time to read through one of my first edits of the book.

My good friend and fellow triathlete Janet Lynch for reading through my book and giving her expertise.

28566794R00114

Made in the USA
San Bernardino, CA
02 January 2016